TOM WATSON

DOWNSIZING

How I lost 8 stone, reversed my diabetes and regained my health

KYLE BOOKS
LONDON

An Hachette UK Company
www.hachette.co.uk

First published in Great Britain in 2020 by
Kyle Books, an imprint of Kyle Cathie Ltd
Carmelite House
50 Victoria Embankment
London EC4Y 0DZ
www.kylebooks.co.uk

ISBN: 978 0 85783 833 9

Publisher: Joanna Copestick
Editorial Director: Judith Hannam
Editorial Assistant: Florence Filose
Design and typesetting: Peter Ward
Production: Caroline Alberti

A Cataloguing in Publication record for this title is available
from the British Library.

Printed and bound in the UK

10 9 8 7 6 5 4 3

To Jo Dalton, who made me find the time
to live for the people I love.

Contents

Contents

Prologue

On a chilly evening in December 2012 I attended a festive get-together hosted by a former colleague. Leanne Johnstone had worked alongside Gordon Brown in Downing Street for a couple of years – she'd organised his diary – but had relocated to the United States in 2010. She returned to England every Christmas to spend time with her extended family, though, and this particular year had also decided to organise a meet-up in a central London pub for her old Westminster friends.

The place was full of familiar faces, including a clutch of MPs and civil servants. With a pint of Guinness in one hand and a pork pie in the other, I found myself chatting with a workmate's husband, a consultant dermatologist by the name of Dr Sunil Chopra. I had never really spoken to him at length before, but I found him to be a really interesting and engaging character. He told me all about his research work, notably the development of an ointment to treat basal cell carcinoma, one of the world's most prevalent cancers.

'All being well, it'll have the potential to save thousands of lives,' he said.

'That's incredible,' I replied. 'Sounds like you've made a great breakthrough.'

Sunil then quizzed me about various parliamentary

goings-on, including my involvement in the News International phone-hacking inquiry that had taken place that year.

'Loved the way you took the Murdochs to task.' He smiled. He was referring to the Commons' Culture, Media and Sport select committee meeting that I'd spearheaded in the midst of the scandal.

'I've got a copy of the final *News of the World* framed on my office wall at Westminster,' I said, smiling back. 'Can't say that I miss it.'

Dr Chopra and I continued chatting for a few minutes, until our conversation hit a slight lull. I noticed him nervously running his hand through his hair, as if something was vexing him.

'Everything all right?' I asked.

'Listen, Tom, I've really enjoyed speaking with you,' he said, lowering his voice to a near-whisper, 'but there's something else I'd like to discuss, if you don't mind.'

'Go ahead,' I replied, assuming that he was going to ask me about the Tory government's cuts to medical research, or something along those lines.

'There's no easy way of saying this,' he went on, taking a deep breath, 'but I have a feeling you may be diabetic.'

What the hell… yelled a voice in my head as I took a few moments to process this bolt from the blue. Sunil, meanwhile, shifted uneasily from one foot to the other.

'I know I may be stepping out of line here,' he said, 'but I'm just a little worried that you could—'

'Hang on a minute,' I interrupted, a little testily, 'you're assuming that just by looking at me? I mean, I know I'm overweight, but...'

'I'm a medic, Tom, and I just happen to know a little bit about type 2 diabetes,' he said, offering me a sympathetic smile. 'My hunch could be wrong – I hope it is – but I really think you need to get yourself checked out.'

'Maybe we should go somewhere a little more private,' I replied, mindful of eavesdroppers in this pub full of revellers. I'd been a parliamentarian long enough to know how quickly gossip could spread through Westminster.

So, in a quiet corner away from the hubbub, Sunil outlined the various 'markers' that had triggered his diabetes radar. He began, perhaps unsurprisingly, with my chunky frame, which, as per usual, was clad in a black, baggy suit. I rarely weighed myself, but I guessed I was edging toward 22 stone (140 kilos).

I cringed slightly as Sunil suggested that my solid pot belly could be an indicator of excess deep abdominal body fat – so-called 'visceral' fat – a small amount of which normally surrounds vital organs such as the liver and pancreas. This condition often pointed toward insulin insensitivity, he explained, which was a precursor to developing type 2 diabetes.

My frequent trips to the loo that evening (probably averaging about three per hour) had also given him cause for concern – I hadn't realised he was keeping a toilet tally, I told him – and he was worried about my general appearance, too, blushing slightly as he described me as 'a little bit clammy-looking' (he was spot on, to be fair; I never went anywhere without a pocket handkerchief to dab my damp brow).

While Sunil reeled off a litany of diabetes indicators, as the strains of 'Jingle Bell Rock' floated across the pub, I actually felt a little sorry for him. Informing a relative stranger that he might be suffering with a serious, life-changing disease can't have been an easy thing to do in the circumstances.

'Mince pie, anyone?' said Leanne, smiling, as she approached us with a large platter of festive nibbles. I took this as my cue to bring our chat to a close.

'Certainly not the kind of conversation I expected to have at a Christmas party, Sunil,' I said, firmly shaking his hand, 'but maybe I should thank you for being so honest.'

'Just get yourself booked in for that blood test,' he replied, perhaps relieved that I hadn't told him to back off and mind his own bloody business, 'and if I were you, I'd do it sooner rather than later.'

In February 2013, having spent a few weeks mulling over this bombshell, I found myself perched on the edge of a chair in the Westminster surgery of Dr Shaukat Nazeer, awaiting the results of my blood test. My GP, in his early seventies, with a shock of greyish-white hair, scanned the all-important printout, nodded his head and confirmed that yes, with my blood glucose levels coming in at 6.7 mmol/l (millimoles per litre), I did indeed have type

2 diabetes. I had officially joined the ranks of nearly three million sufferers in the UK.

'I must say, you don't seem very surprised, Tom,' he said, peering at me over his wire-rimmed spectacles.

'No I'm not, really,' I responded, with a shrug of the shoulders. 'I hadn't exactly come here expecting good news.'

Indeed, in the lead-up to my appointment I'd consulted a wide variety of books, articles and websites relating to type 2 diabetes. Although I was very wary of presupposition and self-diagnosis, there was no doubting that many of my own signs and symptoms had tallied with those that I'd read about: a constant thirst, an uncontrollable appetite and poor sleep quality, to name but a few.

Dr Nazeer, with typical pragmatism, then outlined the disease that, in all likelihood, I'd probably been suffering since I was in my thirties. Type 2 diabetes, he told me, was a long-term metabolic disorder that occurred when someone was severely insulin-resistant, or when their pancreas stopped producing enough of it.

'Insulin is a hormone that helps your cells to absorb glucose, or blood sugar,' he said. 'If it's lacking, or if you don't respond well to it, too much glucose stays in the blood, and not enough reaches the body's cells. And it's that deficiency that makes you feel tired and hungry.'

'That makes sense, I guess,' I said.

'But what you need to realise, Tom, is that diabetes is a very serious condition,' he added. 'Raised blood sugars can increase the risk of strokes and cardiovascular disease, and can cause kidney, nerve and eye damage, so it's really important you keep this under control.'

Given these circumstances, I'd have to get used to monitoring my blood sugar, which would be measured in two ways. Firstly, Dr Nazeer would regularly check my long-term glucose levels via the haemoglobin A1c (HbA1c) test, a basic but effective method that would ascertain how I was managing my condition. Secondly, I could also monitor things on a daily basis myself, using a finger-prick and test strips.

Dr Nazeer then wrote out a prescription for a powerful drug called metformin, which, all being well, would help to regulate my blood sugar levels, thus easing my symptoms and slowing down the disease's progress. He also assigned me to a dedicated diabetes nurse, who I'd visit for regular check-ups and weigh-ins, and referred me to a consultant endocrinologist, who'd help me to gain a better understanding of the illness. In addition, I'd receive one-to-one advice from a specialist nutritionist, who'd assess and address my dietary habits.

I left the surgery and took a taxi back to my Vauxhall flat, feeling totally and utterly deflated. While the diagnosis hadn't come as a surprise, the prognosis had knocked me sideways. I had been given the distinct impression that my type 2 diabetes was irreversible, that I'd be popping pills for the rest of my days and that I'd be shackled with this chronic and debilitating condition for ever. I felt like I'd been dished out a life sentence.

Introduction

There is a tendency in these polarised times to believe everything, or to believe nothing. These pages are an account of what worked for me on the journey to losing 100lb (45 kilos), reducing my blood pressure and reversing my type 2 diabetes. I began 2018 several stones heavier, and I left the year feeling so much lighter, in so many ways. It was a journey that began with three books written by Dr Michael Mosley, Dr Aseem Malhotra and Dave Asprey, and which exploded into an obsessional amateur interest in nutritional science and cellular biology.

To those who may think that *Downsizing* is a blueprint, I apologise in advance, because it's not. All I can do is tell you how I changed my life in 12 months, what led me to my darkest moments and what helped me to see the light. You must find your own route to success, though, and you must develop your own rules and rituals. My weight-loss journey worked for me, but it's not for everyone, and prior to embarking on any low-carb, high-fat (LCHF) diet you should be checked out by your GP, particularly if you are on insulin or are taking other medications.

I also need to emphasise that, whenever I reference diabetes in this book, it will invariably relate to type 2 diabetes. Type 1 diabetes is an autoimmune disease which results in the body destroying the cells in the pancreas that produce insulin and, as a result, it cannot be reversed or put into remission. It is an important distinction to make.

I don't claim to be an expert in the field, either — I'd prefer to describe myself as an obsessive amateur biohacker — but, when it comes to type 2 diabetes, I'm living proof that it can be managed (or even reversed) through a combination of diet and exercise. With this in mind, I'm committed to telling my story with honesty and candour, and I'm keen to challenge the orthodoxies at the very heart of public policy.

Some will no doubt condemn me for what I have to say; after all, I broke the nutritional guidelines endorsed by my own government. To them, I can only say that I did it to the best of my ability by reading relevant studies and research and, whenever I needed clarification, I sought advice from people with a scientific background. Others may not want to believe my articulations because they challenge the findings of people who are far more qualified than me. I am sorry if I annoy or offend anyone in this respect but, putting it simply, I can only speak from my own personal experience, and this particular route proved successful for me.

In the end, to understand the science of weight loss you have to enter ferocious global arguments being waged between clinicians, governments and food conglomerates over many continents. And you have to deconstruct some very powerful axioms that are so fundamental to our lives that they determine what we choose to put into our bodies.

I broke the most powerful food rule of all: the one that said that fat is bad for us. Incredibly, increasing my saturated fat intake helped me to break a thirty-year sugar habit. I am a sugar addict, you see. If I'd continued consuming the sucrose (and other sugars) that sustained three decades of cravings, I could well have been dead by now. And that's the other thing you learn when you are a hundred pounds lighter, and mercifully sugar-free: sucrose is the most powerful drug in the world. And when this toxin eventually breaks your pancreas, the fat produced in your liver from starchy carbohydrates continues the damage by effectively strangling your organs.

Let me emphasise that again: I am a sugar addict. I believe I will die if I resume this dependency, and for that reason I still employ the approach of a former drug user to create a basic daily discipline of eating food and buying food. And as I've journeyed toward a healthier life, I've begun to understand the all-pervasiveness of the 'Big Sugar' economy. The corporations that run the global system of production and consumption – Kellogg's, Coca-Cola, Pepsi, that's you – are using every ruse they can to hold up reform of the system.

If Vladimir Putin had silently poisoned four million British citizens, we'd be at war with Russia. Yet these huge conglomerates – which I've taken to calling the 'Global Sugar Industrial Complex' (or GSIC) – have helped create a societal tolerance of sugar that has done just that, and more. Of the three million-plus type 2 diabetics, two million of those currently medicated by the NHS have an entirely reversible condition. Now that I've experienced this physical and emotional turnaround for myself, I feel like I've found a new goal in life: Remission for All.

But the health journey for me has also been politically instructive. There's a golden rule of politics: the more harm an industry inflicts, the greater the lobbying spend. When a former House of Commons intern sent me a Christmas card from her new role at British Sugar, I knew I was on to something. The more I learned about the techniques used by the GSIC, the more I realised that the sugar lobby is the biggest and most powerful of all. They literally hack our brains.

The biggest gain from losing a third of my body mass was the most unexpected: I've got my brain back. A thick fog has been lifted. I can recall facts quicker and my concentration is deeper and longer. I can pay attention in meetings more than before. I have more patience. I feel more compassionate. I say this because if two million of the UK's 3.4 million type 2 diabetes sufferers can achieve similar mental gains through quitting sugar, then we can significantly lift the productive capacity of the nation. Our international cognitive punch can be accelerated.

So what is stopping people transforming their lives? Contrary to the reflexive commentators in the national press, it's not sloth and laziness. There isn't a simple answer to why, as a nation, we've staggered into a public health crisis of our own making; but I do believe that one of the likeliest reasons is global sugar's all-pervasive marketing.

They make Russia's fake news factories look like amateurs. Not only do the GSIC hack our brains, they try to manipulate our emotions. Those Michael Jackson concerts you went to as a kid? Pepsi sponsored them because an executive probably wanted our childhood memories to be synonymous with soda-pop. And Coca-Cola's marketing plan explicitly states that they seek to 'inspire moments of optimism and happiness'. This is why they sponsor big sporting events, not the surgical wards that amputate the toes and feet of British men and women week after week due to sugar-related conditions. For the millions of us who are predisposed to sugar intolerance and insulin resistance, this is manifestly not the case.

If you're reading this book it's likely that you're concerned about your weight, or your hypertension, or your high blood-glucose readings. Perhaps you're feeling anxious about your health, and are fearful for the future.

Please don't panic. It is eminently possible that, through nutritional change and a slight increase in exercise, you can actually transform your health. And if you have type 2 diabetes or pre-diabetes, you may even be able to reverse your condition or significantly improve it. I am testament to that.

At 52 years old, and having transformed my health, the pursuit of a long and purposeful life carries far greater significance for me than when I was a hedonistic young man. I want to live another half-century, and I want it to be fulfilling. I have effected changes in my life to make that outcome more likely and, because I hold a position of relative influence in the public arena, I want others to be allowed that same opportunity. Ultimately, I'm keen to encourage others with type 2 diabetes to experience the many benefits of remission. As a Member of Parliament I often hear the phrase 'take back control'. That's what I've done, and I'd love others to be able to do the same with regard to their own bodies. I want them to have the joy of transformation. I want them to feel stronger and smarter.

Since I revealed my diabetes diagnosis, back in September 2018, I have been moved and inspired by the extraordinary public response and support for my personal battle. Hundreds of people have contacted me through emails and via my social media channels to say how they have struggled with their health and well-being, just like me. So many people have been in the same boat as me, beset with feelings of guilt, denial and helplessness in the face of being diagnosed with a deadly serious, potentially life-limiting condition. That's why I felt compelled to write this book: to inform others with type 2 diabetes that you have nothing to be ashamed of, and that you are so far from being powerless.

On the one hand, *Downsizing* is a polemic on how global sugar is wrecking our society, and is a call to arms for a Remission for All movement. On the other hand, it is the shared insight of a middle-aged fat bloke nicknamed Tommy Two Dinners who lost 100 pounds in a year, who found the will to exercise and who rediscovered his health and happiness.

And who still eats bacon and eggs for breakfast.

CHAPTER ONE
Tipping the Scales

We Watsons loved our food and, thanks to my mum (or 'mom' if you hail from the West Midlands), we certainly got our fair share of it. While the family coffers weren't exactly overflowing – my parents both worked for the council, and didn't earn a fortune – Mom budgeted very well and always ensured that her brood enjoyed plenty of good grub.

Our Sunday lunches were a weekly institution. While Mom got everything prepared at home, Dad would take me, my brother and my sister to a working men's club, the Habberley, where he'd sink two or three pints with his mates as we drank Coke, munched Quavers and played on the fruit machines. We would make our way back home at about three o'clock, to be greeted with a meal of either steak and kidney pie served up with creamy mash and peas, or roast beef and Yorkshire puds swathed in home-made gravy.

Despite being stuffed to the gills – Mom's portions were massive – we'd invariably make room for pudding. There would be a chorus of '*mmmmmm*'s as Mom, wearing oven mitts, brought in crowd-pleasing desserts like syrup sponge served with custard or, if the ice-cream van happened to come down our road that afternoon, dollops of Mr Whippy. Legend had it that Margaret Thatcher helped to invent that particular brand of ice cream when she was a chemist in the 1950s.

'That woman stole your school milk, Tom, but she also gave you Mr Whippy,' my dad would say.

My parents split up in the late seventies, sadly, but the Sunday lunches continued with my stepdad Barry at the table. Indeed, he loved Mom's apple pie so much that he persuaded her to commercialise production.

'D'you know what, Linda, people would pay good money for that pie,' he'd often say, wiping the crumbs from his mouth with the back of his hand. 'No one makes pastry like you.'

'Thanks, Barry, love,' she'd reply, beaming.

He wasn't wrong. Soon Mom would be selling her sweet and savoury offerings to our local Berni Inn, based at the Riverboat restaurant on Blackwell Street. The place was the height of sophistication in 1980s Kidderminster, boasting a huge all-you-can-eat salad bar and housing one of the few Atari 'Pong' arcade games in the area.

Mom's culinary repertoire became even more adventurous when she subscribed to *Supercook* magazine, and my brother, sister and I would return home from school to be greeted with the aroma of her freshly baked creations. Her showpiece Battenberg cake, with its pink 'n' yellow chequerboard, blanketed in thick marzipan, looked almost too good to eat.

Unfortunately, there was no such food heaven at school. In the early 1980s, the Tory-run Herefordshire and Worcestershire County Council had sacked the dinner ladies at King Charles I Comprehensive and, in the name of progress, had decided to privatise the service. Almost overnight, canteen-cooked meals were dropped from our lunchtime menu, and were replaced with reheated fast food including hot dogs, hamburgers and doughnuts. Those pupils entitled to free school dinners (me included) were given yellow meal tokens worth 45p, which only stretched to a battered sausage and a handful of chips. Unimpressed, I'd often flog my token for 40p, sneak out of the school gates and scamper over to Captain Cod's on Station Hill. There, I'd hand over my ill-gotten gains for a 'Scholar's Special': a steaming parcel of sausage and chips (35p) plus a potato scallop (5p). Mrs Thatcher might well have been proud of my entrepreneurial spirit, but Mom was having none of it.

'Tom, you'll get into bother,' she muttered one day after some local busybody had spied me queuing outside the chippy in my school uniform. 'If they end up taking your tokens away, you'll be using your pocket money instead.'

In spite of my hearty appetite, I was an averagely built teenager (playing lots of schoolboy rugby probably helped to keep me slim). I really started to pile on the weight in my early twenties, however, having become addicted to junk food and cheap beer while studying politics at Hull University. There, I'd found myself developing a fondness for beer and burgers, and a weakness for the city's drinking dens and takeaways. A bellyful of Skol in the John McCarthy Bar was often followed by a chicken madras from the venerable Ray's Place. I would frequently be accompanied by my housemate, Neil Codling, a great lad who, incidentally, would one day end up playing keyboards for Suede.

Fried breakfasts were the order of the day in our *Young Ones*-esque student digs, comprising platefuls of greasy eggs and gristly sausages, served up with baked beans, HP sauce and a stack of buttered white bread. My role as president of the Student Union wasn't exactly conducive to a healthy lifestyle, either, since the events I helped to organise – gigs, ceilidhs and freshers' festivities – were often very boozy affairs. As time progressed, and my penchant for anything fatty, fizzy or sweet persisted, I ballooned rapidly and was forced to upsize my baggy, beige Marks & Spencer cardigans to Large. And then to Extra Large.

It was around that time that I received a stern talking-to from the university's GP. I had visited her surgery for some flu medication, and while I'd been there she'd decided to measure my height and weight.

'You're fifteen and a half stone,' she'd said, grimacing as I'd stepped onto the scales. 'You do realise that's in the obese BMI range, don't you?'

I confessed that I'd never heard of this 'BMI', or body mass index, which prompted the GP to explain its implications and question my fitness and nutrition.

'Putting it simply, Tom, you need to eat less, drink less and move more,' said the doc.

No one had ever upbraided me about my weight before – maybe they'd not seen it as their place to do so – yet I felt suitably admonished and embarrassed enough to take action. First and foremost, I enrolled at the campus sports centre, signing up for some circuit training sessions and occasionally using the cycling and rowing machines. Then I had a stab at moderating my food intake, albeit rather half-heartedly. For two or three months I only ate fried breakfasts at weekends, and I replaced my carry-out curries with microwaved 'healthy options' (although the portions of the latter were so tiny I often ate two). While I wasn't prepared to give up alcohol – Dr Killjoy wasn't going to deny me that – I compromised by substituting my pints of lager with halves.

Despite all this, my weight remained static, and I couldn't say that I felt any healthier. Resigned to the fact that I was innately hefty – and assuming I was naturally 'big-boned' – I quit the gym, binned my diet and resumed my old habits. *Sod that for a lark*, I thought.

'Steady on, Tom, no one's going to take it off you,' I remember my housemate Simon Shott saying as I wolfed down a Friday night doner kebab, sluicing it down with a 'full-fat' Coke.

'You know what, I could eat another one of those,' I'd said, smiling, as I polished off every morsel of my meat 'n' carb fix, convincing myself that I simply needed more fuel than my slimmer, sprightlier friends.

As it transpired, I quit university earlier than planned to take up a role with my beloved Labour Party as a youth development officer. Left-wing politics had run through my family like letters in a stick of rock and, for me, the lure of a job at the Walworth Road HQ had been impossible to resist. My parents were long-time party members and activists – Dad had served as a local councillor in our home town of Kidderminster – and our kitchen was always alive with debate and discussion regarding the issues of the day. Whether it was the Watergate scandal in the United States, or Margaret Thatcher coming to power in the United Kingdom, the Watson clan (including my younger brother Dan and my little sister Meg) were well-informed on the issues of the day.

Around the time of the Three-Day Week – and during one of the many power cuts we experienced during the electricity shortages – I vividly remember lying on my top bunk, eating a banana sandwich in the dark.

'Why do the lights keep going off, Dan, and why is Mom walking around with a candle?' I asked my brother, who always kipped beneath me on the bottom bunk.

'She says it's because that horrid Mr Heath won't pay the miners enough money,' came his reply.

I was an activist from an early age. I remember when I was seven years old, during the 1974 general election, helping out my parents by delivering Labour Party leaflets through letter boxes, collecting polling numbers at the nearby Franche Primary School and pasting electoral registers onto display boards with Copydex. I became completely enthralled by the procedures and mechanics of the voting system, whether it was the Get Out the Vote (a.k.a. 'GOTV') battles between local volunteers, or the excitement of the final count in the town hall. I loved observing the candidates as they nervously watched ballot papers being sorted into piles, always crossing my fingers for the person sporting the big red rosette.

As it happened, the youth development job was my second role at Walworth Road. I had actually secured my first position with the Party in my late teens, having just left sixth form. Fancying a taste of London life – I'd become a tad bored with life in provincial Kidderminster – I'd applied for a £5,400-a-year trainee library assistant post, and had been thrilled to get the job. Being a computer nerd worked in my favour, I think. Although I'd spent many an hour playing *Manic Miner* and *Jet Set Willy* on my Sinclair ZX Spectrum, I'd taught myself some elementary coding, too. This fitted in with the library's plans to invest in a computerised database for lendings, returns and renewals ('It's the future, Tom,' I was told at the time).

My remit also included collating press clippings from the daily selection of tabloids and broadsheets, and typing up documents for various MPs, councillors and activists. On my very first day, in the winter of 1984, I found myself sharing a lift with party leader Neil Kinnock and his deputy Roy Hattersley, but was far too star-struck and tongue-tied to utter a single 'Hello' or 'Good morning'. Further down the line I'd receive a handwritten letter from the great Tony Benn (whom my dad hero-worshipped) thanking me sincerely for assisting him with the cuttings service. I treasured it for years.

Not long after my start date, I was taken out for lunch by a senior member of staff, Ted Higgins. He took me to the nearby Tankard pub in Walworth Road to sample their legendary 40p sausage baguette and, being on the executive committee of the Campaign for Real Ale, he introduced me to Bass beer. I fell asleep at my desk that afternoon – not the last time that would happen to me in my working life – but I made amends the next day, joining in with the staff aerobics session that regularly took place in the top-floor boardroom.

Walworth Road was abuzz with activity in those days. In 1985, singer Billy Bragg had launched the Red Wedge musicians' collective to attract younger voters to the Labour Party, and I was asked to support the promotions team, who were organising a variety of concerts and events featuring artists like the Communards, Elvis Costello and the Attractions, the Style Council and Madness. For me, this was both a pleasure and a privilege – I was an *NME*-reading indie-music aficionado – and, in January 1986, I remember being in my element as I watched Billy, Paul Weller and an avant-garde duo called Frank Chickens performing at the Birmingham Odeon. That evening's compère (who also happened to work in the Red Wedge office) was the inimitable 'Porky the Poet', also known as comedian Phill Jupitus. We often chatted about music at Labour Party HQ – he knew loads of up-and-coming bands – and I remember him handing me a shiny new Housemartins badge as we chinwagged by the photo-copier.

I bid farewell to Walworth Road after the 1987 general election to take up a job with the Save the Children charity, before embarking upon a short-lived stint as an advertising agency account executive. Hull University subsequently intervened, and then – four years after my librarian role, and carrying three extra stone (19 kilos) – I found myself back at Labour HQ.

'Wow, Tom, you've put on some timber,' commented a party activist who'd known me back in the day. 'What happened, eh? Did you overdose on fish and chips up north?'

As I smiled through gritted teeth, I remember thinking *Oh, do fuck off, you cheeky bastard...*

I graduated from youth development officer to deputy general election coordinator (my seven-year-old self would have been so impressed), working under legendary campaigns manager and bon viveur Fraser Kemp. Then, operating from the new Labour Party headquarters in Millbank, I became part of the well-oiled machine that helped to propel Tony Blair into 10 Downing Street on 1 May 1997.

However, when the dust settled, and when promises of a more influential post-election role failed to materialise, I decided to apply for the position of national political officer with the Amalgamated Engineering and Electrical Union (AEEU). Based in the Kent town of Hayes, it was a hands-on campaigning role that included a great deal of weekend work and late-night meetings. The camaraderie and comradeship was second to none, though. One of my closest colleagues was the incomparable Bill Tynan, a regional officer in their Glasgow office who, shortly after

I'd joined the union, had taken great pleasure in introducing me to a 250-strong convention of electricians and engineers in his native city.

'This is Tom Watson,' he'd announced on stage, throwing me a sideways glance. 'He's from our head office in London, England. He used to work for Tony Blair, at Labour HQ, in Millbank, London. Today he's come up to Glasgow, Scotland to tell us how to do our politics. Over to you, Tom…'

Cheers for that, Bill, I thought, as boos and jeers (good-natured, I hoped) floated across the auditorium.

I survived the meeting – just – and afterwards Bill and his fellow activists, Gerry Leonard and Allan Cameron, whisked me over to a city-centre pub to sample some local hospitality. There was a significant drinks culture in union circles – they worked hard, and definitely played hard – and it was only after downing pints of beer for eight hours solid that I was allowed to stagger back to my city-centre hotel.

Back at our Hayes HQ I met a no-nonsense Yorkshirewoman called Siobhan, who was based in the estates department. I had actually first met her at a somewhat bizarre work night out – she'd beaten me in an arm-wrestling contest at an Elvis impersonators' restaurant in Streatham – and we'd immediately hit it off. I recall inviting Siobhan over to my Bromley flat for our first evening meal together, and spending the afternoon cleaning my kitchen from top to bottom; I don't think she'd have been impressed by the columns of empty Stella Artois cans, or the leaning tower of Domino's pizza boxes.

We were soon engaged to be married, and began to

make plans for a July 2000 wedding in a Kidderminster church. I got myself measured up for a smart two-piece suit – it was so expensive I had to borrow the money for it – and Siobhan found herself a nice bridal gown. Throughout the spring, however, I had so many lads' nights out (including a five-day stag do in Barcelona) that I had a shock when I rocked up for the final suit fitting. All my partying had taken its toll and, as I surveyed my reflection in the mirror, all I saw was my gut hanging over the waistband and my chest bursting out of the shirt.

'The wedding's only a month away,' I groaned. 'There's *no way* I can turn up looking like this.'

I arrived at work the next day in full-on panic mode, asking my colleagues if they had any emergency weight-loss advice. Coming to my rescue was my PA, Cathy Pearce, who delved into her desk drawer and handed me a photocopy of the cabbage soup diet.

'If it's a quick fix you want, Tom, this'll do the trick,' she whispered, folding it over as if it were subject to the Official Secrets Act. 'I won't lie, it tastes horrible and it's a little, erm, unsociable, but some of the staff have sworn by it.'

'You're a star, Cathy,' I replied, before heading off to the local Asda to plunder their stocks of savoy cabbage and vegetable Oxo cubes.

My workmate wasn't wrong. While I rapidly lost weight on this bland, boring diet – I whittled myself down to 17 stone (108 kilos) – it proved to be insufferable not only for yours truly, but also for those friends, family and colleagues who had the misfortune to share confined spaces with me. Let's be honest: I reeked from both ends. At home I went through about twenty canisters of Air Wick, and at work Cathy would casually leave packets of mints on my desk to nullify my cabbage-scented belches.

All this effort had the desired effect, though – thank God – since I just about managed to squeeze into my posh suit on the Big Day. Unsurprisingly, by the end of our honeymoon in Bali I'd regained much of the weight I'd shed. After weeks of fasting on watery soup, I was desperate to eat some proper food.

'I never want to see another cabbage again,' I said to Siobhan as I tackled a huge plateful of pad thai.

Physically, my wife and I were like chalk and cheese, so much so that some friends playfully dubbed us 'Laurel and Hardy'. Siobhan was a slender, sporty fitness fanatic who had plans to train as a boxing instructor, while I was a lardy, lethargic couch potato who got breathless walking to the corner shop. And, as time went on, my eating habits began to spiral out of control. A prime example of this occurred during a weekend visit to some friends in Oxford. On the Saturday evening they rustled up a delicious beef casserole, followed by a dessert of home-made Bakewell tart and custard, which they knew was a particular favourite of mine. After coffee and mints, we spent a pleasant few hours chatting, drinking and listening to music, but when they finally went upstairs to bed – and with my stomach rumbling non-stop

– I felt compelled to make a detour. I crept into my friends' kitchen, quietly opened their fridge and ogled the left-over Bakewell tart.

I'll just have a tiny sliver for supper, I thought, as I grabbed a jammy wedge and dipped it in the jug of cold custard. *One's not going to hurt, is it?*

Before I knew it, however, I found myself polishing off the remaining three slices too, leaving behind just a smattering of pastry crumbs. Any sense of dignity, propriety and restraint vanished as I succumbed to an intense and irrepressible urge to sate my hunger. I didn't enjoy it. I didn't even taste it. I just had to have it.

I then exited the kitchen and trudged upstairs, wondering how I was going to explain myself in the morning. *A-ha, they've got a pet cat*, I thought. *I'll blame him...*

My Bakewell-tart binge shocked me into taking action, though – my overeating was getting ridiculous – and within days I'd signed up to Weight Watchers (now WW) online. I was far too busy (and far too ashamed) to attend the group sessions at a local community centre, so the organisation's recently launched website seemed a more viable option. However, despite sticking rigidly to the programme for a few months – I meticulously planned my meals, and obsessively counted my calories – I only shed a few paltry pounds. For whatever reason, Weight Watchers and I were incompatible.

'God knows where I'm going wrong,' I remember lamenting to Siobhan. It was as puzzling as it was dispiriting.

*

In February 2001, at the age of 34, I decided to run for a seat in parliament. I had been encouraged to put my name forward by a handful of AEEU members in my prospective constituency, West Bromwich East; evidently they'd been impressed with the work that I'd done on the Rover task force, a government-organised group that had helped to prevent the closure of the Birmingham-based car plant. The prospect of becoming an MP was not a decision I'd taken lightly – I loved my union job, and I also had Siobhan to consider – but in the end it just seemed like the right thing to do. My former mentor, Fraser Kemp, had sensed my anxiety and, over a pint one night, had proffered some words of wisdom.

'If you want to change things in society and make a difference, Tom, you have to seize every opportunity,' he'd said.

'It's a bit of a leap in the dark, though, mate...' I'd replied.

'Maybe it is. But I reckon you should go for it.'

On Thursday 7 June 2001 I was duly elected as an MP, as part of Tony Blair's second administration, and my whole world changed overnight. While I relished my new life as a politician – it was an absolute honour to represent my constituents, and to serve alongside such luminaries as Dennis Skinner and Margaret Beckett – I found my work schedule immensely challenging. In order to fulfil my parliamentary and constituency commitments, I spent most weeks shuttling between Westminster and the West Midlands, attending a cavalcade of meetings, briefings, surgeries and conferences. No day was ever the same, but the vast majority began extremely early and ended very late (occasionally beyond Big Ben's midnight chimes if there was a vital House of Commons vote). Not only did these long hours and erratic schedules disrupt my sleep patterns and heighten my blood pressure, they also played havoc with my eating habits.

With neither the time to do a weekly shop at the local Tesco, nor the inclination to rustle up a home-cooked meal, the food cupboards in my Bromley flat – which I'd maintained as my London base – remained sparse. The contents of my fridge usually amounted to a packet of roast ham (often past its sell-by date), a litre of full-fat milk and a few cans of Guinness.

I always stocked up with breakfast cereals, though – a healthy and nutritious way to start the day, I reckoned – and would habitually grab myself a bowl or two of Kellogg's Cornflakes or, when I was feeling particularly peckish, a supersized serving of Scott's Porage Oats, into which I'd stir a banana and a dessertspoon of honey. If I was ever pressed for time, though, I'd grab a couple (yes, two) bacon sandwiches in the Commons' canteen, traditionally referred to by MPs as the 'Members' Tea Room'. Comprising thick rashers of bacon, encased in soft, white, buttered bread, these butties were the best I'd ever tasted.

A couple of hours later, when my mid-morning hunger pangs inevitably took hold, I'd gladly help myself to the plates of biscuits that were always laid out in meeting rooms in the Commons. More refined colleagues than I might have nibbled at a Hobnob, or munched a couple of Jaffa Cakes, but I'd regularly scoff the whole lot. I was acutely aware that I was committing a social faux pas – I tried to ignore all the tuts and the raised eyebrows – but, as time went by, I realised that my need for satiation outweighed any sense of decorum.

Lunch in the Tea Room would usually comprise a large portion of pie and mash or, if we had a sitting session on a Friday, a plateful of fish and chips. Whenever the afternoon lethargy set in (much to my shame, I'd sometimes find myself nodding off at my desk) a chunky KitKat usually did the trick, giving me a much-needed sugar hit and acting as a timely, albeit temporary, pick-me-up.

I wonder if other MPs feel as exhausted as I do? I'd ask myself as I aimed the wrapper into the rubbish bin.

Then, later in the evening, I'd often avail myself of a takeaway.

'Hello again, Tom,' my friendly delivery driver would say with a grin as he handed over my large stuffed-crust Meat Feast, with a side of BBQ chicken wings and the requisite can of pop. If I was ever feeling double-hungry I'd opt for their 2-for-1 deal – *treat yourself, Tom, you've had a hard day* – knowing that I could polish off any leftovers the following morning.

An hour later, once the gratification had faded and the fatigue had descended, I'd find myself slumped on the sofa, trying my damnedest to stay awake for *Newsnight*. Feeling guilty and gluttonous, I'd question my lack of willpower and discipline – *why the hell can't I stop filling my face?* – and, by and large, I'd generally reach the same conclusion: here

I was, a supposedly intelligent individual (a Member of Parliament, no less) who couldn't control his own body. Junk food had me in its thrall.

My bulky frame and my hearty appetite soon earned me the nickname of 'Tommy Two-Dinners' around the Palace of Westminster. This soubriquet originated from a food- and booze-fest that took place at the legendary Gay Hussar in Soho, a Hungarian restaurant that was favoured by the Left, back in the day when politics (and journalism) was fuelled by mountains of food and rivers of alcohol. On that particular afternoon I lunched with *Guardian* journalist Kevin Maguire and *Tribune* editor Mark Seddon, putting the world to rights and sharing Westminster gossip while we enjoyed a meal of roast duck, washed down with bottles of Merlot. After a couple of hours, Kevin bade us farewell to file an article back in the office, and Mark and I decided to stay in the restaurant and continue through to dinner.

At about five o'clock we both began to flag, so the Gay Hussar's manager, John Wrobel, allowed us to sneak off for a recuperative nap in the Tom Driberg suite – a private dining room – where he put up two camp beds for us, and folded up tablecloths for us to use as makeshift pillows. After about half an hour he returned to revive us with hot towels and glasses of champagne, and we staggered downstairs for our second sitting of food and drink. News of our overindulgence soon spread, however. A few days later an item in the *Evening Standard* appeared, referring to me as 'Tommy Two-Dinners', and the nickname duly stuck.

'Here he comes, Tommy Two-Dinners,' my fellow MPs would say, sniggering, as I queued up for lunch in the Tea Room.

Colleagues constantly ribbed me about my lack of sartorial style, too. For reasons of comfort, I'd often sport a custom-made, baggy black suit teamed up with an untucked shirt and a loosened tie. Following one particular Commons debate, I was informed by Mark Tami MP – a good friend of mine – that I was 'the only bloke who could make a five-hundred-quid suit look like a fifty-quid suit.'

The political 'lobby' journalists had their own take on my distinctive appearance, too, and would regularly describe me in print as a 'bruiser', a 'fixer' or a 'henchman', portraying me as a straight-talking, hard-nosed tough guy. While I found this characterisation quite amusing, I also thought it somewhat misplaced; yes, I possessed a rash (and occasionally reckless) streak, and yes, I could occasionally be a bit mouthy, but no more so than most of my Commons colleagues. I certainly didn't recognise the 'bovver-boy' badass featured in their parliamentary profiles and sketches.

The *Guardian*'s political cartoonist, Steve Bell, did his utmost to perpetuate this image, too, adding to the sense that I was this brutish, thuggish MP. Many politicians found themselves at the rough end of his pen – former prime minister John Major was given a particularly hard time – but his caricatures of yours truly were especially excoriating. He took delight in depicting me as a grotesquely overweight monster, bursting out of my black suit and glowering behind my heavy-rimmed spectacles, more often than not surrounded by disproportionately skinny Labour Party colleagues. I generally took it in fairly good humour, ever-conscious that a thick skin was compulsory in order to survive in the merciless world of politics. That said, I did find it a bit rich that the satirist himself wasn't remotely sylphlike.

In spite of my health and lifestyle challenges I made decent progress in government – Tony Blair appointed me a government whip in 2004 and, two years later, I was promoted to junior defence minister – and, on the whole, I felt pretty confident and comfortable within the House of Commons environs. From a professional perspective I tried not to let my weight issues hold me back or curb my ambition and, among colleagues of all ranks, I never allowed myself to feel inferior. At Westminster I'd happily chair meetings and deliver speeches without an iota of inhibition, and at party conferences and rallies I'd invariably be the last man standing, swapping stories with delegates, sharing pints with reporters and belting out the Kaiser Chiefs' 'Ruby' on the karaoke.

There were instances, though, when my weight issues brought about some awkward situations at work, none more so than on my first day at the Ministry of Defence in Whitehall. The maximum-security entrance comprised a tall, glass, cylindrical structure featuring two concave doors. The first door would open in front of you, allowing you to step inside the tube and process your ID, before the second concave door opened, enabling you to walk out and continue into the building. But it didn't quite happen that way for me. As soon as I entered the tube I set off a piercing alarm, which caused both doors to clamp tightly shut.

I was trapped inside for a few moments, with the sirens still wailing, before a red-faced security guard came over to release the door and free the new minister. Much to my embarrassment, it transpired that the system had detected that two people had entered, not one, and had essentially gone into lockdown (the MOD would later have to reset and reconfigure the system in order to specially accommodate me). I couldn't have imagined a less auspicious, and more humiliating, start to my new job.

I had also experienced a similarly toe-curling moment when the Labour Party announced its anti-obesity 'healthy living' strategy. I was on frontbench duty in the Commons that particular day, sitting beside the comparatively lithe Secretary of State for Health, Alan Johnson, as he outlined our plans to provide overweight people with incentives to change their diet and to participate in exercise. As I squirmed in my seat, blushing profusely, I could see a few Tory MPs nudging each other and smirking in my direction. God knows what those TV viewers tuning in to *News at Ten* later that evening must have thought.

'Well, the big fella next to Johnson hasn't exactly read the brief, has he?' I imagined Dave from Doncaster sniggering, with good reason. 'I bet he's dodged a few salads in his time…'

From that day onward I did my utmost to steer clear of

any committees or announcements associated with health or obesity, since my presence within that context was simply farcical.

Once I'd exceeded the twenty-stone mark, my activity levels nosedived. The half-mile walk to my workplace was nigh on impossible – I'd since relocated to a new flat in central London – so most mornings I hailed a cab to the Carriage Gates entrance. So indolent did I feel, however, that I was hardly able to look the driver in the eye as I handed over the minimum fare for this two-minute journey.

Upon arrival at the Commons I'd head straight for the lift, because the steep staircase to my office was a complete non-starter (I couldn't manage the descent, either). When it came to organising meeting venues – particularly in the afternoon, when my lethargy hit hard – I'd ask my staff to book rooms in Westminster to avoid walking any kind of distance. Indeed, I often found myself trying to duck out of any meetings that were scheduled off-site, even those within a stone's throw of parliament; if this proved to be unavoidable, I'd have no option but to flag down another taxi, and yet again let the cab take the flab.

Even more troubling for me, however, was the way my obesity affected the quality time I spent at home with my young family. Sadly, Siobhan and I had decided to separate in September 2010 – the aggressive press intrusion during the News International phone-hacking inquiry was partly to blame, prompting my wife to relocate to the Yorkshire

Dales – but we remained firm friends and co-parents, happily sharing the care of our son Malachy (born in 2005) and our daughter Saoirse, three years her brother's junior. We agreed that I'd look after the children on alternate weekends, in addition to half of the school holidays. Occasionally the kids had no option but to join me on the road, tagging along with me to various political meetings and conferences. I clearly remember Saoirse falling asleep during one of my speeches ('The Future of the Labour Party', I seem to recall) although in the circumstances I couldn't really blame her; it wasn't the most exciting speech I'd ever delivered.

While I liked to think I was a caring and capable father (aside from the political events, we had lots of fun times together), I was acutely aware that my obesity often held me back. I couldn't help Malachy hone his football skills, for example, as I didn't possess the stamina to go in nets or take a corner. I never took Saoirse to the local swimming baths, either, for fear of not being able to complete a length, and because I lacked the confidence to wear trunks in public. Indoors, there were occasions when I could barely engage my son and daughter in conversation, or read them a bedtime story, because I felt so drained and exhausted. I constantly felt that I was letting my lovely children down – there was a distinct lack of 'presence' on my part – and it broke my heart.

'Why are you falling asleep, Daddy?' Saoirse would ask, midway through a rendition of our favourite Spike Milligan poem, 'On The Ning Nang Nong'.

'I'm just a little bit tired tonight, Sershy-Wershy,' I'd reply, mustering up a drowsy smile as my daughter's big blue eyes stared up at me.

So, despite my perpetual fatigue and my mushrooming girth, I spent my entire forties – in fact, I wasted my entire forties – sweeping my health concerns under the carpet. I was caught up in a mire of dread and denial, too embarrassed to discuss my predicament with my loved ones, and too preoccupied to attend 'well man' check-ups with my GP. Indeed, I always resisted the temptation to google my symptoms, for fear of what I might discover. Something told me that typing 'incessant hunger', 'morbidly obese', 'raging thirst' and 'excessive fatigue' into a search engine would doubtless generate a message to GO DIRECTLY TO DOCTOR, which I simply didn't have the time or the inclination to do.

Instead, like many middle-aged men before me, I effectively ignored the warnings, donned the blinkers and hoped that my ailments would simply fade away. Even in February 2013, when Dr Nazeer finally diagnosed me with type 2 diabetes, I spent the ensuing three months purposely concealing my illness from my family. I was loath to cause them any upset or alarm – especially my children and my parents – and I was also racked with shame and embarrassment. The way I viewed it, my poor lifestyle choices had got me into this unholy mess, and my failure to act on the omens and flag up my symptoms had been foolhardy in the extreme. It was my fault, and my fault only, that I had jeopardised my long-term health. There was still a huge amount of disbelief on my part, too; the prospect of lifelong diabetes was so scary and unfathomable that I could hardly bear to contemplate it myself, let alone talk it through with others.

Eventually I'd drum up the courage to speak with my family and friends – cue a succession of frank and honest conversations – and, to a man and woman, they couldn't have been more supportive. My sister Meg, a qualified nurse, was particularly sensitive to my issues, and was keen to nudge me in the right direction.

'Without wanting to frighten you, Tom, you really do need to get this under control. It's such a serious condition. Listen to your doctor, of course, but you always know where I am if you need me.'

'Cheers, sis, I appreciate that…'

Afraid that my illness might be perceived as a weakness in the Commons bear pit, I initially kept my Westminster colleagues out of the loop, too. Throughout 2013 and 2014 I never breathed a word to a single soul; but, as it turned out, it was through my own carelessness that I was eventually rumbled.

'Here, you left these on your desk,' whispered my office manager, Karie Murphy, one morning, as she handed me a foil strip of metformin while I turned a deeper shade of puce. Being a former nurse herself, my colleague recognised my medication and understood its significance.

'To be fair, Tom, I've been worried about you for a while,' she said, 'but I didn't think it was my place to pry.

I'm so glad you're addressing things, though. Time to keep off those chocolate Hobnobs, eh?'

2015 proved to be extremely gruelling, work-wise. The springtime general election campaign, with Labour challenger Ed Miliband contesting Tory leader David Cameron, saw me visiting over one hundred constituencies up and down the UK. My public profile had risen in the wake of the phone-hacking inquiry, and as such I was asked to coordinate so-called 'member mobilisation' (drumming up support, basically) in key parliamentary seats that Labour had to win or defend. On average, I'd visit four or five constituencies per day, adhering to a punishing schedule that saw me delivering town centre speeches, giving media interviews, posing for photos with Labour candidates and knocking on doors to canvass voters.

I was often assisted by a team of local activists and, on occasion, by a left-leaning celebrity; the comedian Eddie Izzard, whom I admired very much, lent his support in a number of constituencies, including Amber Valley and Northampton North. All this to-ing and fro-ing was no good for my health and well-being, though, and for five weeks my diet largely comprised full English breakfasts in hotels, and takeaway burgers in cars.

Things would only get busier. The following September, having attended a string of hustings from Brighton in the south to Edinburgh in the north, I was elected deputy leader of the Labour Party – succeeding Harriet Harman – on the same day that Jeremy Corbyn was chosen to replace Ed Miliband at the helm.

'It's my role to unify the party, hold things together and make it work in difficult times,' was my message to those who'd voted me in.

Amid all this politicking I continued to have regular diabetes check-ups and, having been referred by Dr Nazeer, also managed to squeeze in an appointment with an NHS nutritionist in central London. It proved to be one of the most humiliating half-hours of my life. As I sat in her consultation room, she quizzed me about my food and drink intake – I gave her an honest summary of my daily excesses – before introducing me to the Department of Health's 'Eatwell Plate'. This laminated pie chart, divided into colour-coded segments, illustrated the government's official recommendations in relation to a wholesome, balanced diet.

'Now this is probably the best way to explain it to you,' she said, a little condescendingly, before placing a large red plate on her desk. Upon it lay various shiny, plastic foodstuffs, including a chicken drumstick, a cheese wedge, a bread roll, a carrot and a pineapple. The kind that Malachy and Saoirse had once pretended to cook on the hob of their Toys R Us kiddies' kitchen.

The nutritionist explained that the Eatwell guidelines endorsed a healthy and varied diet that included five portions of fruit and vegetables a day, with a meal plan based around starchy carbohydrates like potato, bread, rice or pasta. Fat, especially saturated fat, should be reduced — it raised cholesterol, apparently, which could increase the risk of heart disease — and foods high in sugar were to be restricted, too.

As she outlined each segment, she pointed to the corresponding toy ('bread for carbohydrate... chicken for protein... pineapple for fruit...') and a little part of me curled up and died. Here I was, Tom Watson, Member of Parliament, deputy leader of the Labour Party, ardent campaigner for justice, being made to feel like I was appearing on some mid-morning CBeebies show. With typical British propriety, though, I just smiled, nodded and — once the consultation ended — thanked her kindly for all her help and guidance.

How on earth has it come to this? I said to myself as I traipsed out of the clinic, consumed with self-pity.

CHAPTER TWO

Inspired

Living with a morbidly obese junk-food addict can't have been easy. A couple of years before my diabetes diagnosis, I'd struck up a relationship with Steph — she worked for a trade union — and we'd moved into a terraced house in the West Midlands town of Cradley Heath. I would catch the train up from Westminster most Thursday evenings (I often had constituency duties the following day) and, more often than not, Steph would drive over to collect me from the station since the half-mile, seven-minute walk was way beyond my capabilities.

My weight frequently brought about some awkward moments in our household. I remember breaking numerous G Plan dining room chairs, the wooden frames buckling and splintering under the strain of my 22-stone bulk. Once, to my eternal shame, I even cracked the bath, the plastic base caving in as I attempted to haul myself out. Steph had a healthy relationship with food, and had generally tried her best to curb my wayward appetite, but her efforts were often in vain. She would despair as the kitchen cupboards were emptied within days of the Tesco 'big shop', shaking her head as she watched me demolish a jumbo bar of Dairy Milk or an entire tube of cheese and onion Pringles.

'Tom, can't you just have a couple of chunks instead of

the whole bar?' she'd ask, but I'd usually be too busy filling my face to answer. For me, wolfing down the entire block of chocolate was a physical and physiological compulsion: I couldn't *not* eat it all. I continued to be troubled by this lack of restraint, though, and would often ask Steph to hide my sweet and savoury treats so as to remove the temptation. Her most effective hiding place, I later learned, was at the bottom of a stack of saucepans.

I also remember her once encouraging me to bake some 'guilt-free' flapjacks — made with oats, nuts and coconut oil — to use as an alternative snacking option. I ended up devouring all eight of them in one go (my mindset was 'but they're *good for me*, right?') and afterwards I felt so nauseous that I almost threw up.

My brazen eating habits continued when we stepped out of the front door, too. If we ever visited our local McDonald's Drive-Thru, I'd order two cheeseburgers instead of one Big Mac, purely because they were easier to grasp as I scoffed them at the wheel (waiting until we got home to eat them was never an option). Once, Steph met me for lunch in a city centre café, only to find me staring blankly at my laptop while helping myself to some leftover rainbow cake that another customer had abandoned on the adjacent table.

'Tom!' she'd hissed, as a passing waitress looked on disdainfully. 'What the hell are you playing at?'

'Oh my God, I'm so sorry,' I'd replied, aghast, before explaining that my cake-pilfering had been utterly involuntary. I'd genuinely not known what I was doing.

Recalling this faux pas would always make me wince with embarrassment.

Throughout our time together, such lapses in concentration were commonplace. Steph would often remark that I seemed dizzy and disorientated or, as she put it, somewhat 'disengaged from the present'. She would talk about me 'zoning out' of conversations, so much so that if she had a list of questions to ask me, she would pose the most important one first, because by the third I'd have totally switched off. Neither of us knew it then, of course, but this detached listlessness was most likely a result of diabetes-related hypoglycaemia (commonly referred to as a 'hypo'), triggered by a sharp drop in my blood sugar levels.

My relationship with food improved marginally, however, once I'd received my T2D diagnosis, and once Dr Nazeer had referred me on to the NHS nutritionist. Urged to follow the Eatwell Plate guidelines, and keen to do things by the book, I adhered to much of her advice. I began to monitor my portion sizes, measuring out my carbohydrates using small kitchen scales like she'd suggested. I remember, at breakfast time, carefully weighing out 20g of dry porridge oats – which probably equated to a fifth of my usual supersized serving – and wondering how on earth that was going to sustain me until lunchtime. More often than not it didn't, and I'd find myself indulging in elevenses, and loading up with a croissant or two.

Furthermore, I tried to limit my consumption of sugary foods, cutting back on my favourite cakes and biscuits. I also stocked up my kitchen cupboards with fresh, low-calorie produce and – as the nutritionist had suggested – rustling up the occasional home-made meal instead of relying on a takeaway. I was a fairly proficient cook when I put my mind to it, although I always tended to opt for super-elaborate Yotam Ottolenghi or Madhur Jaffrey offerings, which invariably required a long list of exotic ingredients, and commandeered two hours of my time. The end result was usually delicious (Steph was very impressed) but I really should have focused my energy on building a repertoire of simple, easy-to-prepare everyday meals, in order to bring more consistency to my dining habits. With me, though, it was all or nothing.

Despite implementing these changes, and despite trying to follow the standard guidelines, my weight seemed to plateau rather than plummet and, disappointingly, I continued to experience overwhelming carb and sugar cravings. My willpower wobbled and wavered – typically when I was in my London flat, following a long day at work – and I'd often end up yielding to a late-night toasted sandwich and a bottle of Fanta Orange, before nodding off on the sofa.

One positive development, though, was the emergence of a certain mindfulness with regard to my eating, and a nascent realisation of the relationship between food and physiology. Although I was still unable to resist the temptation of that toastie and that fizzy drink, I felt myself becoming more aware of my actions, and more conscious of how certain foodstuffs affected me. With this, though, came a certain frustration at my powerlessness. It seems I had identified carbs and sugar as the enemy, but hadn't yet found the ammunition to vanquish them.

On Thursday 23 June 2016, the day of the UK's European Union referendum, I was as fat, as tired and as unfit as ever. A fortnight earlier, however, I'd mustered up enough energy to deliver a speech in Granary Square, near King's Cross, for the 'Britain Stronger in Europe' campaign. Spandau Ballet's Gary Kemp – like myself, a staunch Remainer – introduced me on the stage, in front of hundreds of supporters. Meanwhile, a couple of miles away, Sir Bob Geldof traded insults with Nigel Farage on the Thames, each having commandeered cruiser boats for their rival campaigns.

'There is an economic case, a social case, a patriotic case and a political case for us to remain in the EU,' I said to the crowd gathered in the square. 'And there is also a Labour case. Cooperation. Peaceful existence. International solidarity. These are Labour values.'

By my side on voting day was my 11-year-old son Malachy. His head teacher had kindly given him special dispensation to take the day off school – so long as he did his homework – and had agreed with my view that he'd benefit greatly from witnessing democracy in action at such close quarters. My son had jumped at the chance to spend this most momentous of occasions with his dad in London. He had developed a genuine interest in politics (he was fascinated by polls and elections, not unlike my childhood self) and had closely followed the referendum run-up. We attended various media appointments that morning, paying visits to all the pop-up television studios located on the green outside Westminster. My son, no doubt feeling slightly star-struck, was thrilled to meet household-name presenters like Sky's Adam Boulton and the BBC's David Dimbleby.

'It's clear that Britain is better off in Europe,' I asserted in interview after interview, as my son watched proudly from the wings. Our time together was precious, and it was so nice to have him around.

Malachy and I spent the rest of the day mobilising the vote on the official Remain bus, alongside my colleague Keir Starmer. We also squeezed in a visit to the Labour Party's campaign HQ, something that I was keen to do for two reasons. Firstly, I wanted to hook up with its coordinator, Patrick Heneghan, as well as the staff who'd worked so tirelessly over the previous few months. Secondly, and more selfishly, I wanted to indulge in the pizza and chocolate that every campaign office worth its salt had on offer. As I munched on a deep-pan pepperoni, I remember seeing the nervous expressions on my colleagues' faces as the exit polls began to filter through. The Brexit result was going to be tighter than we'd ever imagined.

The final stop for me and my mini-helper was my Westminster office, which was housed in the same tower as Big Ben. There, we made ourselves a little dad-and-son den, placing the sofa cushions on the floor, surrounding ourselves with snacks and drinks and watching the results coming in from the various counts across the UK. We channel-hopped between the three main news sources until, as the clock struck 3 a.m., we could no longer keep our eyes open. A few hours later we woke up to the shock news, delivered by Mr Dimbleby, that Leave had prevailed, taking 52 per cent of the vote.

'I just can't believe it, Dad,' said Malachy, glumly shaking his head.

'You and me both,' I replied.

Later that morning, feeling utterly crestfallen at this outcome (and suffering the after-effects of a 24-hour carb and sugar binge), I dropped Malachy off with his mum. And, as the day panned out, it soon became pretty apparent that I'd have to delay my scheduled trip to the Glastonbury Festival. Steph and I had initially planned to catch a late-afternoon train from Paddington but, amid all this political tumult, we decided instead to set off the following day. In hindsight, I should have perhaps cancelled the entire jaunt – my workload had multiplied overnight – but I didn't want to let my partner down. It was going to be her first ever trip to this world-famous music-fest, and I didn't want to be seen as a party pooper.

Within hours of arriving in Somerset, and having set up camp and dumped our sleeping gear, we decided to drown my post-referendum sorrows by going on a spectacular drinking spree. Downing can upon can of cider, I watched Adele crooning her greatest hits repertoire on the main stage, followed by a few bands in the Left Field tent (where we happened to bump into my pal Billy Bragg), and soon enough the previous day's trauma was shoved to the back of my mind. Any thoughts of healthy eating were cast aside, too, as I did the rounds of the street food vendors, feasting on pulled-pork buns and Belgian chocolate churros.

Sometime after midnight, Steph and I found ourselves stumbling through a muddy field, following signs for the Silent Disco tent. There, we drank and danced until 5 a.m., giggling at each other as we threw some serious shapes to the tunes pumping through our headphones. At one point I decided to capture our revelling on Snapchat, uploading a goofy-grinned selfie and captioning it with 'Silent Disco!' alongside the bespectacled 'nerd' emoji. In hindsight, perhaps not the most rational decision ever made by a sitting Member of Parliament.

I awoke the following day feeling dry-mouthed and fuzzy-headed, my joints aching after the previous night's excesses. Fumbling for my mobile phone to check the time, I happened to notice that there were stacks and stacks of missed calls and messages.

'Get your arse back to London, Tom,' one text read. 'It's all kicking off here...'

'Seems like you're having a blast at Glasto!' said another. 'Rave on dude!'

A little confused, I immediately went online. According

to various news sites, the Labour Party was in turmoil, Jeremy Corbyn having sacked Shadow Foreign Secretary Hilary Benn from the front bench amid rumours of a leadership coup, which had led to reports of senior colleagues threatening to resign in protest. Making matters a whole lot worse for me, however, was the fact that a handful of newspapers had published images of yours truly standing in the middle of a Glastonbury field, sporting baggy clothes and muddy wellies, and clasping a can of Thatchers cider.

'Tom Watson enjoys Glastonbury disco as civil war erupts in Labour Party,' gloated one headline, as a #FindTomWatson hashtag trended on Twitter. Not only that – and this explained the 'rave on' text – screenshots of my drunken Snapchat posts had been bandied around the internet for all to see. In the circumstances, this didn't look good. In fact, it looked absolutely bloody dreadful.

You are an utter dick, Watson... I remember thinking to myself as Steph and I gathered our belongings and made a premature exit. We had only been at Glasto for 12 hours.

A couple of press photographers were there to greet me at Castle Cary station just before 10 a.m., gleefully snapping away as I shambled along the platform, missing my train by seconds. According to the timetable, the next London-bound service was due in two and a half hours' time, so we had no choice but to plant ourselves on a bench, in the middle of nowhere, and sit it out.

I remember Len McCluskey, boss of the Unite union, ringing my mobile and giving me one hell of an ear-bashing.

With my head banging, and my blood sugars crashing, I didn't have the energy to return fire.

'Len, could you please shout more quietly?' I replied.

A few days later, back in Westminster, I took myself away from the political wrangling (and the relentless Glasto-related piss-taking) to attend my monthly diabetes check-up. I was dreading the outcome, to be honest; my weekend partying, as well as my referendum-related comfort eating, had no doubt played havoc with my blood sugar levels and had definitely added more wobble to my waistline.

'Right, let's get you weighed,' said Maggie Jones, a very experienced and uncompromising practice nurse. Her expression was a mixture of concern and disappointment as the scales settled at a point just past the 22-stone (140-kilo) mark.

'You've actually *gained* three kilograms since last month,' tutted Maggie. 'That's not great, is it?'

'No, it's not,' I said, feeling thoroughly ashamed of myself as I dismounted the scales. Maggie went quiet for a few moments before asking me to take a seat.

'Now, I'm sorry if this sounds a little blunt, Tom, but have you ever considered weight-loss surgery?' she asked. 'I mean, I know it's seen as a last resort but, well, judging by your age, weight and BMI range, the NHS would probably agree to a gastric band or bariatric surgery. But only if you wanted it, that is.'

'Let me think about it, Maggie,' I said, with a doleful shake of the head.

As it happened, I'd previously discussed the pros and cons of these procedures with my sister Meg, and had reached the conclusion that – despite it being a viable option for obese patients like me – it wasn't a route I wanted to pursue. Having looked into the various procedures, I reckoned there were less risky and more humane methods of weight control than one of these highly invasive surgical interventions.

However, in spite of my scepticism, the fact that my diabetes nurse had even chosen to broach the subject was pretty sobering in itself, and marked yet another low point for me. I was at the top end of the morbidly obese range on the BMI scale, which is just about as bad as it gets. By suggesting the most drastic of solutions, she was flagging up the gravity of my condition. It was a warning light, a wake-up call.

That night I had a long moan to Meg over the phone, explaining how demoralised I'd felt following the check-up, and – despite my recent lapses – how disillusioned I'd become with the NHS Eatwell shtick. Despite following the official guidelines as best I could, and despite heeding the professional advice meted out, for months my weight had stubbornly refused to budge from the 285–300-pound (129–136-kilo) range. It was frustrating beyond belief.

'I'm losing faith in it all, Meg,' I told her. 'Calorie counting, portion sizes, it's just not working for me. I just don't feel as though I'm getting anywhere.'

'Maybe you need to look at some other options,' she said. 'There's plenty of information out there, Tom, and plenty of alternatives to investigate.'

Having always relished a challenge, and being something of a science geek, I started to learn all I could about diabetes-related nutrition, and began to explore other ways in which I could mend my ailing body. Tellingly, I decided to conduct my own private research into my condition rather than discussing it with fellow sufferers. My social circle contained a number of middle-aged men who'd been diagnosed with type 2 diabetes, but I'd purposely avoided having any man-to-man conversations with them. There was no doubting that I felt a certain shame about the illness, and was embarrassed to share my symptoms and coping strategies with anyone else, lest I appeared weak or inferior. I allowed myself to suffer in silence and solitude, almost like I was punishing myself.

So, whenever I had any spare time on my hands – on a Yorkshire-bound train to collect my kids, or in a post-conference hotel room – I'd pore over a book I'd bought, or a research paper I'd printed, carefully marking the most interesting and thought-provoking passages with highlighter pens and Post-it notes.

At the top of my reading list was *The 8-Week Blood Sugar Diet*, written by the acclaimed science journalist Dr Michael Mosley. 'How to prevent and reverse type 2 diabetes (and stay off medicine)' it claimed on the front cover. 'Lose weight fast and reprogramme your body.'

I read it on Steph's mum's Kindle during a weekend

break in Malaga – Sheila often advised me on food-related matters – and I devoured every single page. The author, who had himself been diagnosed with type 2 diabetes in his forties, offered a short, sharp and effective solution to blood sugar issues, asserting that metabolic syndrome (the umbrella term for a cluster of conditions that put you at risk of heart attacks, strokes and type 2 diabetes) could be controlled, and even reversed, through diet as opposed to drugs. He advocated a rapid weight-loss programme as the best way to combat type 2 diabetes, which meant adhering to a low-calorie, low-carbohydrate, Mediterranean-style eating plan. Starchy carbohydrates, he suggested, caused a rapid increase in blood sugar levels, and triggered the crashes that led to hunger pangs.

'Standard nutritional advice is under attack like never before,' he wrote. 'The age-old instruction to "eat low fat" has been seriously undermined by numerous studies which show that such a regime is rarely effective and people who go on it rarely stick to it. The trouble is that when people cut out fat they get hungry, so they switch to eating cheap and sugary carbs, one of the main causes of the dietary disasters we have today.'

Having become increasingly cynical about the big red Eatwell Plate, I found it illuminating to discover that his doctrine largely eschewed the standard nutritional advice offered by the NHS, which was still telling me to graze on pasta, rice and bread.

'This is a tasty and healthy way of living,' explained Dr Mosley, while extolling the virtues of his diet plan. 'It is low in starchy, easily digestible carbs, but packed full of disease-fighting vitamins and flavonoids. It is rich in olive oil, fish, nuts, fruit and vegetables, but also contains lots of lovely things that down the years we have been told not to eat, such as full-fat yoghurt and eggs.'

Full-fat yoghurt? Eggs? Sounds good to me... I thought.

Dr Mosley's work on VLCDs (very-low-calorie diets) appeared to be based on robust science, and had been significantly influenced by the work of Roy Taylor, Professor of Medicine and Metabolism at the University of Newcastle. This renowned academic had discovered that type 2 diabetes was related to excess amounts of fat in the liver and pancreas – i.e. around the waist – and that weight loss removed this harmful fat. This in turn enabled these organs to start working normally, thus allowing insulin to do its job properly.

Professor Taylor's 2011 clinical study (sometimes referred to as the 'Newcastle Diet') investigated the potential benefits of an ultra-low-calorie eating plan for those with T2D. Eleven patients with the condition were put under close supervision and had their intake of food – largely comprising soups, shakes and vegetables – reduced to 800 calories per day for a period of eight weeks. It turned out that, three months later, seven of those patients had shed fat from around the liver and pancreas, had reported a normalisation in their blood glucose levels, and were effectively in remission from their type 2 diabetes. (Further down the line, Professor Taylor's study would be scaled up and published in *The Lancet* under the auspices of DiRECT, the Diabetes Remission Clinical Trial.)

Reading Dr Mosley's book, and learning about the Newcastle Diet, proved to be a eureka! moment for me. It was a revelation to discover that type 2 diabetes did not have to be a chronic, lifelong condition, that it was not inevitably progressive and that, in some cases, it was entirely reversible. Following two years of doom, gloom and pessimism, I felt my mind had been opened, and that I was finally able to cling onto some real hope for the future. I genuinely felt that I'd taken a step, albeit a baby step, toward tackling my own personal, health-related conundrum, one that, for years, had remained unsolved.

When I returned home to England, buoyed with optimism, I penned a rather gauche, Adrian Mole-style letter to Dr Nazeer, describing how thrilled I'd been to read Professor Taylor's findings (I'd even attached a hard copy of his study), and outlining my determination to find the drive and energy to turn my own life around.

To learn that I have a metabolic syndrome that may be reversible is a revelation, I wrote. *I would like to concentrate on doing just that, reversing the condition, with your guidance and support... the question is, as the study points out, do I have the motivation?*

My reasons for writing the letter were twofold. Firstly, to almost show off to my GP, to demonstrate to him that I'd done my homework, and that I was now approaching my condition in a studious and scholarly manner. Secondly (and perhaps subconsciously) I was exposing my vulnerability; I'd become deeply worried about my deteriorating health, and

I needed him to realise exactly how eager I was to find a solution.

Dr Nazeer responded to my missive with characteristic kindness. Other GPs might have felt rather affronted that I was effectively questioning their advice, and exploring other options, but with him this wasn't the case. Indeed, he even invited me over to his surgery for a chat, where we had a mature conversation about my potential choices and considerations. He took care to reiterate public health dietary guidelines – as an NHS GP, it was incumbent on him to do so – but at the same time he pledged his continued support. I inferred from our conversation that, if I ever succeeded in my quest to lose weight, get healthy and ditch my medication (even via unconventional means), Dr Nazeer would be thrilled for me.

'Thank you so much for listening,' I said, shaking his hand. 'It means a lot.'

My voracious – nay, obsessive – reading continued apace during the autumn and winter of 2016, despite a huge increase in my parliamentary workload. That October, following a reshuffle, I'd been appointed Shadow Secretary of State for Culture, Media and Sport. I was thrilled to bits to take on this role. The brief was right up my street, and I relished getting my teeth into issues such as the planned Sky takeover by Fox, the proposed closures of grassroots music venues and fairer ticketing for football fans.

'You? Shadow secretary for *sport*?' texted one of my old rugby teammates once he'd heard the news. 'They mustn't have seen you in action on the pitch, Tom...'

I did manage to fit in some extra-curricular reading, though, much of it prompted by the extensive footnotes and references in *The 8-Week Blood Sugar Diet*. Dr Mosley's own bibliography had helpfully pointed me to other books, articles and scientific studies and, slowly but surely, I began to gain a much broader understanding of diabetes-related health and nutrition.

I was also inspired to research old-school diabetes and dietary advice (once a nerd, always a nerd) and spent much of my spare time trawling through various charity shops and second-hand booksellers, and placing late-night eBay bids for rare and obscure titles. As time went by, I amassed a decent collection of vintage cookery books, social histories and medical directories. Their contents made fascinating reading; I was particularly interested to learn how increased prosperity in Victorian Britain had led to workers eating a low carb diet that was rich in protein and high in fat, including plenty of lard, oysters, haddock and herrings as well as succulent Sunday joints. Breakfasting on bacon and eggs or cold meats and cheese wasn't unusual, either, although that was before Dr Kellogg had begun his campaign for the world to eat corn flakes.

I also managed to lay my hands on a slightly gnarled edition of *The Nicomachean Ethics* by Aristotle. He is known as the 'father of Western philosophy', and his words of wisdom had provided me with a great deal of solace and guidance ever since my university days. I remember taking this old book back to my flat, and being particularly drawn to a quote that pretty much encapsulated my past, present and future challenges.

> *First then this must be noted, that it is the nature of such things to be spoiled by defect and excess; as we see in the case of health and strength (since for the illustration of things which cannot be seen we must use those that can), for excessive training impairs the strength as well as deficient: meat and drink, in like manner, in too great or too small quantities, impair the health: while in due proportion they cause, increase, and preserve it.*

I celebrated my fiftieth birthday on 8 January 2017, and marked this milestone by throwing a huge knees-up for friends and colleagues at the Rivoli Ballroom in south-east London. The only authentic 1950s ballroom still standing in the city, it had retained all its original vintage decor – velvet chairs, flock wallpaper, glitterballs – and, to me, seemed the ideal party venue. I booked a brilliant covers band to entertain us all, Rockaoke, whose repertoire of seventies and eighties classics, like Bryan Adams' 'Summer of '69', got the dancefloor bouncing (quite literally, in fact, since it was one of those fabulous sprung versions).

I laid on a free bar for the first hour or so to get the party started and to get my guests well oiled – this went down as well as expected – and also put on a giant buffet comprising my favourite sweet and savoury treats. The centrepiece, however, was an enormous cake, fashioned in the shape of a large grey robot sporting my signature black-framed glasses. It was a mickey-take of my geeky nature, reflecting my love of gaming and my admiration for automatons and artificial intelligence.

In attendance that night were many former schoolmates from Kidderminster, as well as a few Hull University pals. Comedian Steve Coogan came along, as did ex-Undertones frontman Feargal Sharkey, both of whom I'd known for some years. Westminster colleagues on the invitation list included fellow MPs Rachel Reeves and Lucy Powell, as well as one of my favourite Labour Party couples, Yvette Cooper and Ed Balls. Ed had not long been voted off *Strictly Come Dancing* and, having been badgered by all and sundry, was persuaded (albeit reluctantly) to re-enact his infamous 'Gangnam Style' dance. Footage of him busting his moves, alongside a laughing Steph, was plastered all over social media the following day.

I got predictably hammered – I'd hit the Guinness with abandon, it being my birthday – and toward the end of the night I ended up clambering on stage with the band to belt out a couple of classics. Nothing, however, had prepared me for Feargal Sharkey grabbing the mic to duet with me on 'Teenage Kicks', his band's biggest hit, and legendary DJ John Peel's all-time favourite record. It was totally and utterly surreal. Had I keeled over with a heart attack at that precise moment (quite likely, considering the state of my health) I'd have left this world a happy man.

Now that would have been one hell of a cool exit, I thought to myself once I'd returned to my seat at the bar, got my breath back and grabbed myself another drink.

*

The following morning, I woke up in my London flat, nursing the mother of all hangovers, and padded downstairs to the kitchen. I fixed myself a glass of water, popped in an Alka-Seltzer and drew up a chair at the table. As I watched the white pill froth to the surface, my mind began to spool through the previous evening's events. Half of me felt elated because the party had gone so well (everyone had a blast, it seemed) but the other half felt distinctly sad and solemn.

My night, unfortunately, had culminated in a silly and childish row with Steph in which regrettable things had been said. On top of that, the reality of my midlife milestone had finally started to sink in. While it had been great to see so many of my fifty-something contemporaries at the party – some of whom I'd known since childhood – their presence had made me feel a little melancholic. All of them, to a man and a woman, looked fitter, slimmer and younger than me. Every selfie and photo depicted me bursting out of my custom-made blue and black checked suit, my arm draped around friends who were a similar age, but who were half my size.

FIFTY AND FAB! proclaimed one of the many birthday cards that I'd received that night, its huge silver lettering superimposed over an exploding bottle of champagne. *FIFTY AND FAT, more like*, I'd thought to myself as I glumly opened it.

In many ways, though, my five decades so far had given me much to be thankful for. Two beautiful children, whom I loved with every fibre of my body. A close network of family and friends, from Westminster to the West Midlands, whose support and guidance I had always relied on. A fulfilling career in high-echelon politics, the sort that I'd dreamed of since childhood, that had provided me with the opportunity to visit a wealth of interesting places and meet an array of inspirational people.

The only thing missing from a truly rewarding life, of course, was the luxury of good health. And, as I sipped the dregs of my fizzy water, my thoughts drifted to one of my political idols, John Smith, who died of a heart attack in 1994, aged just 55. His family, and the Labour Party movement, had been left utterly bereft by our leader's untimely passing.

'He held conviction without obsession; his principles were for application, not for decoration, and his superb intelligence was for practical use, not for adornment,' said Neil Kinnock in the House of Commons on the day after John's death.

And it was while contemplating this most tragic of losses that a voice seemed to float up from my subconscious. A voice that, whenever it had echoed previously, had been swiftly blocked and muted.

I don't want to die. I really don't want to die.

At well over 22 stone (140 kilos) — the heaviest I'd ever been — perhaps premature death was an inevitability, though. Surely the odds were stacked in favour of Tommy Two-Dinners becoming the next MP to be sent to an early grave. Morbid thoughts began to swirl around my head — the prospect of leaving my beloved kids fatherless; being unable to see Malachy and Saoirse grow up; never meeting my grandchildren – and, much to my surprise, I felt my eyes brimming with tears.

It's time, Tom, continued the voice. *Enough is enough. If you don't address your weight soon, you are actually going to die...*

I removed my specs and blotted my damp cheeks with my pyjama sleeve. I had not felt so emotional and vulnerable in a long time, yet somehow it felt like I'd crossed my personal Rubicon. By confronting my own mortality, and by allowing that deep, dark inner voice to break out, I'd finally found the impetus to reclaim my health and save my life. At last, I'd engaged in an existential discussion with myself that had been submerged, avoided and denied for more than two decades.

One burning question remained, however: just when was I going to commence my big plan, and put all the theory into practice?

I reached for my mobile phone, scrolled through its calendar and hovered over the date of 20 July 2017. The start of the House of Commons' annual summer recess. A fallow period, in parliamentary terms, wherein there'd be no early-morning interviews on the *Today* programme, no late-night votes in the chamber and no working groups or committee meetings in between. A timeframe in which, notwithstanding my ongoing constituency work, I could potentially find some private space in which to get fitter and slimmer.

I took a deep breath, and reached across the kitchen table for a notebook and pen. I turned over a new page, upon which I wrote three words: *Project Weight Loss.*

*

In June 2017, I found myself paying a return visit to the Glastonbury Festival, a fortnight after Theresa May had gained her narrow majority in the general election. This time, though, I was travelling down with my good friend David Wild, since Steph and I had parted company six months previously. Along with a group of fellow music-lovers, my pal and I would be spending the weekend in one of the more sedate areas of Glasto (suitable for old folks like us), but it still promised to be a memorable few days. Nevertheless, as our train rattled through the North Wessex Downs, I made a pledge to be on my best behaviour.

'I can't have a repeat of last year, David,' I said, explaining that – in order to keep out of the tabloids – I'd be keeping a low profile, steering clear of the Silent Disco tent and disabling my Snapchat.

'But you'll still be having a drink with the lads, won't you?' asked my friend.

'Yeah, of course,' I replied.

David wasn't to know, of course, that I'd pencilled in Glasto '17 as my final fling before the commencement of Project Weight Loss. It would, in effect, be the last hurrah before implementing what I hoped would be a transformational lifestyle plan.

I made damned sure that I bid farewell to the 'Old Tom' in style, though. I parked any notions of decorum at the Worthy Farm entrance, whereupon I embarked on a three-day, cider-fuelled bender, with some carb-heavy binge-eating in between. Amid the alcohol haze I managed to catch all three headliners – Radiohead on the Friday, Foo Fighters on the Saturday and Ed Sheeran on the Sunday – although my favourite performances came courtesy of singer Nadine Shah and soul man Craig David, whose brilliant, crowd-pleasing set really entertained the masses. Jarvis Cocker's late-night set of cheesy dance tracks was pretty special, too.

In fact, the whole festival atmosphere was in stark contrast to the previous year's, which had been somewhat subdued following the referendum result, and which had been marred by torrential rainfall. In 2017, however, Glasto-goers were treated to a glorious, sun-baked weekend, and, while the Labour Party had not gained power, it had been a perception-changing election, leaving the mostly left-leaning crowd in good spirits. Indeed, I'd never seen anything like the reception Jeremy Corbyn received before his speech on the Pyramid Stage that Saturday afternoon. The whole place was rammed, and so lengthy were the queues that I was only able to watch him from afar, at the rear of the field. There, I joined in the mass rendition of 'Ooooh, Jeremy Corbyn' that reverberated around Worthy Farm. It would have been rude not to.

Despite my efforts to avoid any controversy that year, I still managed to make the headlines that weekend. I was 'papped' as I tramped through a field while sporting a polo shirt and cut-off trousers combo, topped off with a blue canvas 'newsboy' cap. It wasn't my finest look, to be perfectly honest, and the resulting photographs were unflattering to say the least.

'Deputy Leader Tom Watson is back at Glastonbury and is looking as stylish as ever,' mocked one article.

'He wore espadrilles without any socks while mingling with other festival-goers,' sniped another, as if I'd committed some heinous fashion sin.

David didn't exactly help matters, either.

'You look like the Pillsbury Doughboy,' he chuckled, having spotted the offending photograph in one of the red-tops. I deflected his teasing with a shrug and a grin, as was my wont.

The summer recess couldn't come soon enough.

CHAPTER THREE

Fit for Purpose

At 5.30 a.m. on Monday 7 August 2017, I was awoken by the shrill bleep-bleep-bleeeeeep of the alarm clock in my London flat. I rolled out of bed, wandered into my bathroom, stepped onto the scales and watched the digital display rapidly ascending to 308lb (140 kilos); exactly 22 stone. I then padded over to the sink, brushed my teeth, splashed my face and stared into the mirror.

Day One, I told my reflection. *Bring it on.*

After months of thinking, reading and planning, it was finally time to start afresh. It was, at last, time for me to regain control.

Laid out on my bed was a crisp, white Nike training kit, which I'd soon be wearing in readiness for my first session with a personal trainer. I had bought it on the cheap from my local sports outlet; raiding the XXXL bargain bin was one of the few advantages of being obese, and I'd saved myself a fortune. As for my trainers, I dug out a fifteen-year-old pair of barely worn Otomix that had gathered dust at the back of my wardrobe following a short-lived gym membership. As an added incentive, I also borrowed a Fitbit tracker from my mate Steve Torrance (he'd upgraded to a Garmin running watch) in the hope that, over the forthcoming months, it would help me to plot a nice upward trajectory.

All the conventional wisdom said that a successful weight-loss plan involved 80 per cent diet and 20 per cent exercise, so I knew that – whether I liked it or not – any meaningful lifestyle change would need to incorporate a basic fitness programme. Indeed, increased movement and activity was pretty much essential for those hoping to reverse their type 2 diabetes, as it helped to reduce your short-term and long-term glucose levels, and helped you to use insulin more effectively.

'Insulin resistance, which leads to all sorts of blood sugar problems, often starts with inactivity,' wrote the estimable Dr Michael Mosley on his thebloodsugardiet.com website. 'If you don't use your muscles enough, then over time, fat builds up inside the muscle fibres and insulin resistance develops. The best way to reverse this is to get active.'

For over three decades, my physical shortcomings had thwarted any conventional exercise – even half-mile walks were nigh on impossible – and I'd become part of that wider societal trend that saw people virtually chaining themselves to their desks or sofas, and spending comparatively less time outdoors. I desperately needed to break out of that sedentary existence.

Toward the end of our trip to Glastonbury I'd summoned up the courage to have a heart-to-heart with my mate David about all things exercise-related. He had battled with his own weight issues in the past but having embarked upon a healthy living plan himself, I reckoned he'd be a good sounding board. The ensuing conversation was candid, bordering on brutal, as he reaffirmed what I already knew:

if I was aiming for longevity, I'd have to get my act together and transform my whole lifestyle, from diet to exercise. David then made the suggestion that I should kick-start my new fitness regime with his personal trainer, Clayton. An ex-Special Forces soldier from South Africa, this guy had set up a boxing and martial arts gym in Bermondsey and also offered one-to-one private sessions.

'Clayton's the man to sort you out,' my friend had said as we'd sipped cider in the Theatre Bar. 'He'll show you what to do, and he'll keep an eye on you so you don't keel over.'

'Well that's reassuring, David, but point taken,' I'd replied, feeling both pleased and relieved that I'd plucked up the courage to confide in him. 'I'll call him when I get back to London.'

I turned up a few minutes early for my first appointment with Clayton, feeling somewhat anxious and self-conscious. I looked colossal in my new sports gear – even the XXXL kit was a pretty snug fit – and as I walked through the park gate I pulled down the peak of my baseball cap, worried that I might get recognised by a politics-savvy jogger or dog-walker. Clayton had asked me to meet him at 7.30 a.m. in the children's play area in Kennington Park, a pleasant green space south of the river and not too far from my flat. The specific nature of the venue had intrigued me, but I chose not to question it.

Clayton was already waiting for me as I lumbered over. As wide as he was tall – the proverbial brick outhouse –

he shook my hand, dispatched a cursory nod and opened the gate (David had already warned me that Clayton was a man of few words). As I followed him in – it was deserted at that time of day, thank God – I came over all queasy and nervous. This was new territory for me, since I was miles out of my comfort zone, and I was petrified that I was going to a) fail miserably and b) make a total and utter tit of myself.

We kicked off with some very gentle warm-up exercises like side stretches, knee bends and neck rolls, before Clayton explained why he'd chosen the kiddies' corner as our workout area.

'We're going to do some low-impact, basic-level training to improve your stamina,' he said, 'and this playground equipment's perfect for it. Now, let's see where you're at…'

First of all, Clayton asked me to do as many press-ups as I could. Just the mere request made my blood run cold. I could barely manage one – the utter shame of it – and collapsed in a pathetic heap on the tarmac.

Great start, I thought, feeling totally crushed.

'No worries, Tom,' said Clayton.

He then asked me to do some 45-degree press-ups off a nearby park bench instead and, despite my chest almost caving in, I performed two. Once I'd recovered from this Herculean feat, I was taken to the children's sandpit, where I was instructed to jump on and off its wooden rim, which must have been all of eight inches high.

'Let's have fifteen of those,' said Clayton.

Halfway through, I felt so weak and light-headed I

genuinely thought I was going to faint. For a fleeting moment I considered turning on my heel, absconding from the park, heading to my flat and climbing back into bed.

Things didn't get any easier. Dripping with sweat, I was ushered to a miniature bridge painted in gaudy colours, and was ordered to run across it, to and fro.

Why's that fat bloke staggering around a kids' play area? I imagined puzzled onlookers thinking as they passed me by. *That bridge will collapse if he's not careful...*

I was wheezing like a set of old bagpipes after my mini shuttle run, and had to cling on to a climbing frame as I got my breath back.

'I knew I was unfit, but I didn't realise I was this unfit,' I panted.

'Don't be too hard on yourself,' replied my taskmaster. 'The fact you're here in the first place is an achievement. It gets easier.'

I was under no illusions; I'd always known that personal humiliation and pride-swallowing was going to be a necessary part of this process, especially in the early stages. However, never before had I felt as exposed and as vulnerable as I did in that children's playground. My desire to get healthy superseded any sense of indignity, though, and as I virtually crawled back home to Vauxhall I felt a genuine feeling of elation. Clayton's session had almost killed me (I hadn't even been able to say thank you or goodbye, since I could hardly speak) but I felt certain I was going to return for more of the same the following week. The switch had been flicked.

*

As regards diet and nutrition, Day One heralded the start of a new regime of sorts. I didn't feel quite ready to adhere to a structured plan, or set myself any massive targets, so for the time being I decided to go down a less prescriptive route based on monitoring calorie intake and trying healthier options. Determined to curb my long-term sugar addiction (with my fluctuating glucose levels, this *had* to be my main priority), I made a concerted effort to omit sugary carbohydrates from my diet (so no cakes, biscuits or chocolates) and I tried my best to limit starchy carbs like bread, rice, pasta and potatoes. I endeavoured to drink more water and eat more vegetables, and try to make more home-cooked meals. By forming habits and implementing rules – the most important being 'cut out sugar' – I hoped that I'd encourage certain routines, which would in turn morph into daily rituals.

Yet again, I looked to my old mentor Aristotle for some guidance in this regard, sticking one of his most famous quotations to my fridge door:

We are what we repeatedly do. Excellence, then, is not an act, but a habit.

Next to it I pinned a photograph. I had not long returned from a lovely holiday in Majorca with Siobhan and the kids – now and then we still liked to holiday as a family unit – and she'd quite innocently taken a photo of me diving into the swimming pool, with flab flying in all directions. The resulting image was hideous – I looked like a flying whale – and, as I affixed it with Blu-tack, I knew it would act as the perfect deterrent to any late-night fridge raids.

The morning after my inaugural Kennington Park workout, still feeling slightly weak-kneed and wobbly, I tackled a job that had desperately needed doing for months: a wholesale clear-out of my little kitchen. It was high time to consign all foods containing refined sugar to the green recycling bin, so this meant bidding a final farewell to a variety of sweet snacks (goodbye, my beloved KitKats) as well as my favourite breakfast cereals and muesli bars. I didn't want to do anything in half-measures, so nothing remotely sugary was spared the cull. I almost had to adopt the strict, disciplined approach of a recovering drug user, removing all temptation in order to avoid a perilous relapse.

It seemed to me, having scrutinised their labels, that even many of the supposedly 'savoury' convenience foods in my larder and freezer were laden with sugar (61.2g in a supermarket sweet 'n' sour chicken, no less), so into the bin went a stack of microwaveable meals, shrink-wrapped frozen pizzas, tubs of instant noodles and jars of cooking sauces.

Then it was time to clear the fridge of Guinness and Coca-Cola: the drinks that I'd swigged more than any other in my lifetime, but which had no doubt contributed to my health problems. I piled them up next to the sink, snapped back the ring-pulls and ceremoniously poured the dark brown liquids into the sink, watching them bubble and froth as they disappeared down the plughole. I reckoned I'd miss the stout more than the cola. To me, Guinness was a beautiful drink, was so lovingly made, and was best enjoyed in great company. Now I'd just have to find something else to drink with my pal Paul Latham in the Toucan pub near Soho Square.

As I'd planned to limit my refined carbohydrate – no more tempting, late-night cheese toasties for me – I duly donated the George Foreman Grill to the local charity shop. I had often used it to make two toasted sandwiches in one go, filling them with cheese and ham and gobbling them down in minutes. I chucked away any out-of-date ingredients, too (including a six-year-old bottle of black bean sauce) and donned my yellow Marigolds to scrub all the grease and grime from the fridge, the oven and the cupboards. It was, to all intents and purposes, a cleansing experience; a chance for me to reset the dial and start from zero.

That afternoon, I set aside some time to configure a lifestyle tracker on my phone and computer, which I'd use to measure my food intake and activity levels (I opted for the MyFitnessPal app, which seemed to best suit my needs). It came in really handy as a calorie-counter – I got into a habit of inputting my meals and snacks on a daily basis – and it also enabled me to gauge the 'macros' (macronutrients) of everything I ate, which meant breaking down the proportion of fats, carbs and proteins. My first ever food log comprised the following:

BREAKFAST: two large eggs, one avocado, two slices of wholemeal bread

LUNCH (BISTRO): crab salad, spaghetti carbonara and cheese, mixed salad

DINNER: breaded chicken breast and two rollmop
   herrings

DRINKS (NOT INCLUDING TEA AND WATER): four
   glasses of rosé and one glass of white wine spritzer

In total, that day's intake came in at 2,348 calories, 43 per
cent fat, 33 per cent carbohydrates and 24 per cent protein,
which probably wasn't ideal for me in terms of carb levels.
Just logging this was a significant step, though, because I
soon got into the habit of inputting all my food and drink
into MyFitnessPal, which in turn gave me greater clarity
in relation to calorific values and macronutrient balances.
Weaning myself off that carb-heavy spaghetti carbonara and
that sugar-laden rosé wine wasn't going to be easy, but I was
determined to give it my best shot.

As the month progressed, my outdoor exercise became
more routine and, as my confidence increased, I began to
feel less embarrassed in public. I started to go on lots of
early-morning walks, too, often at the crack of dawn. I
had always been more of a lark than an owl, and two or
three times a week I'd awake at 5.15 a.m., throw on my
kit, strap on my Fitbit and head over to Kennington for a
leisurely stroll, bidding the park-keeper good morning as he
unlocked the iron gate.

In the early days of my weight-loss plan, I set myself
tiny but achievable goals – ambling from Lambeth Bridge
to Waterloo Bridge, for instance, or completing one lap of

Dartmouth Park in West Bromwich – but my lack of fitness meant that I rarely went faster than snail's pace. In the park I'd often find myself being overtaken by a toddler in a toy car, or a pensioner on a walking-frame.

'*C'mon, Tom, keep going,*' I'd say, urging myself on as the sweat poured off me.

Occasionally my pal David would join me on my early-morning promenades in Kennington. Our chats were wide-ranging, encompassing current affairs, science, literature and, more pertinently, our newly found articles on men's health. We offered each other a lot of support (we were both porky middle-aged men embarking on similar journeys) and we'd often engage in friendly, motivational competition although, at around 16 stone (102 kilos), he was much lighter and sprightlier than me.

'Let's walk past five lamp-posts without stopping,' he'd say, striding ahead as I shuffled behind him, struggling to keep up.

As I gradually acclimatised myself to walking, however, I allowed myself to raise my targets and expectations. After a fortnight I was able to walk past six lamp-posts, then seven, and then eight. Soon, I found myself completing a whole lap of the park, triumphantly overtaking the toy cars and the walking-frames. Come late August, I was achieving 5,000 steps per day (my Fitbit would emit a congratulatory bleep when I passed the threshold) and, a month later, I'd doubled that tally. Setting these objectives and meeting my goals gave me such a fantastic buzz.

I reckoned that this target-based competitiveness

probably stemmed from my deep-seated love of video games. This lifelong obsession had started on Christmas Day 1982, when my parents had bought me a Sinclair ZX Spectrum home computer, together with various games cassettes. One of my favourites, *Manic Miner*, was a particularly exacting challenge that involved achieving one level and then the next, and which punished any mistakes by sending you spiralling down to square one. That was almost how I felt when I exercised; if I didn't maintain momentum, and didn't improve incrementally, everything would come crashing down and I'd have to start all over again.

I continued my weekly activity sessions with Clayton, which, as he'd predicted, became far less arduous. The exercises that I'd initially found impossible gradually became tolerable, and then – shock, horror! – they actually became rather enjoyable. It being a very dry and mild autumn, we had plenty of opportunity for outdoor training, and Clayton upped the ante by making me do daily press-ups, standing squats and burpee jumps (I was terrible at the latter, embarrassingly bad, in fact, and grew to loathe the damned things). And while I remained a fat, sweaty bloke, still bursting out of my supersized kit, at least now I was a marginally fitter, fat sweaty bloke.

One morning, during a hydration break, I showed Clayton some phone footage of my kids doing some boxing training. Their mum hailed from a family of keen boxing fans, and Malachy and Saoirse had always shared my in-laws' passion for the sport. And, as my PT watched the video of my daughter punching seven bells out of some vinyl pads, he made a suggestion.

'We could do some boxercise ourselves next session, if you want to mix things up a little,' he said. 'We could film a bit of it, and you could show off to your daughter.'

I paused for a moment, feeling slightly reticent about the whole idea.

'No harm in trying, I suppose,' I replied, finding it hard to visualise myself ducking and diving.

The following week Clayton met me in the park's basketball court, carrying two pairs of boxing gloves and a set of foam pads.

I wish I'd never shown him that video, I thought, fearful that more public humiliation was heading my way.

As I'd suspected, what followed was forty minutes of pure hell. Clayton made me pummel the rectangular pads as hard as I could, while constantly bouncing on my feet, and it was absolutely torturous. My chest heaved, my breath rasped, and I seriously thought I was going to vomit all over the tarmac. Worse still, halfway through the session I happened to be recognised by a passer-by, the first time I'd experienced this in Kennington Park. A bloke in his thirties, walking his young son to school, had clearly clocked who I was (the specs and the waistline probably gave me away) and immediately stopped in his tracks. He whispered something to the boy, perhaps explaining that I was a Labour politician, which prompted the lad to press his little face against the surround netting.

'Hey, Tom, who are you punching?' he yelled. 'My dad wants to know if it's Jeremy Corbyn…'

The cheeky little blighter. I couldn't help but laugh, though, albeit mid-wheeze.

From then on, I saw the father and son regularly passing by the basketball court, usually as I was nearing the end of a boxercise session. The twosome always gave me a friendly wave, which the boy would follow up with some words of encouragement.

'Keep it up, Tom,' he'd say, punching the air. 'You're smashing it!'

I would try to wave back – I quite liked these pep-ups, to be honest – but I was often so jiggered that I could barely lift up the boxing glove.

Though it was hard work, I had lots of fun doing boxercise, and I really liked how it made my body feel so pumped up afterwards. That being said, I had no immediate plans to challenge Anthony Joshua, despite the fact that Tommy 'Two-Dinners' Watson would have made a fabulous ring name.

Kennington Park soon became a huge part of my life, thanks to Clayton, and I grew extremely fond of the place. I regarded it as my own outdoor gym, I suppose, and I loved the feeling of being part of the park community, as just one of the many local residents who used it for pleasure and leisure. I would always smile to myself as groups of joggers or cyclists, especially those of a certain age, passed me by.

Maybe that'll be me one day, I'd think, visualising my slimmer, sportier self.

For me, the benefits were psychological as well as physical; after three decades of sedentary living, it was exhilarating to get myself out into the open air, with the sun on my skin and the wind on my face, and see the outside world in all its vibrancy.

I returned to Westminster in early September, following the parliamentary recess. I had made so much progress since the summer (I was eating more healthily, exercising more regularly and sleeping more soundly) and, as a bonus, I'd shed a few pounds, slowly but surely. This minor weight loss wasn't enough for workmates to notice, though, and to most of my fellow MPs, I was still Tommy Two-Dinners, waddling around in the same big black suit and baggy white shirts. The Commons Tea Room staff must have realised that something was amiss, though, because one of their most regular customers had suddenly stopped popping in for his daily bacon butties and his Friday lunchtime fish 'n' chips (cutting out those butties was purgatory, by the way; they'd been part of my life for fifteen years). The more observant among my colleagues might have also noticed that I was now taking the stairs instead of using lifts, and walking to work instead of hailing a cab.

I did let my office staff into my little secret, though. We were a close-knit bunch, and I thought it only right that they should be privy to Project Weight Loss. Also, for the previous few weeks I'd ploughed a fairly lonely furrow (other than chatting with David and Clayton) and I think part of me was ready to share my thoughts and aspirations with this select coterie of colleagues. In all fairness, two of my team, Jo Dalton and Sarah Goulbourne, had at one time or another (and with admirable politeness and diplomacy) tried to nudge me in the direction of a gym or a salad. Back then, I'd not been ready or willing to heed their advice, but now I'd finally started to ring the changes.

'Good for you, Tom, that's brilliant,' said Jo, when I told her about my plans.

'So impressed,' added Sarah. 'Onward and upward, eh?'

I instructed Jo and Sarah to ensure the other core staff were in the loop, but — since I didn't want to put myself under too much pressure at Westminster, or draw undue attention to myself — I asked them to keep matters within our four walls. They were only too happy to oblige, which I greatly appreciated.

I also asked them to be as flexible as possible with my diary in order to accommodate my morning fitness sessions. In the past, I'd always arrived at the office between 8.30 a.m. and 9.30 a.m. (not that late in Westminster terms, as we often had evening votes and events) and it was common for briefings and meetings to be scheduled around this time, via the electronic diary system used by the whole team. However, now that I'd taken the first steps on my health and fitness journey, and was heading in the right direction, I had no intention of ditching my Kennington Park walks or my exercise regime with Clayton. On certain days, therefore, I'd need an early-doors slot blocking out in the diary, with mid-morning or afternoon spaces ring-fenced for any meetings. The plan was to concentrate on my fitness for an hour, return to my flat to get showered and dressed and report to the office for no later than 10.30 a.m.

Jo and Sarah did their very best to accommodate this but others in the team, who were all vying for my diary time, sometimes forgot. Much to my frustration, I'd discover that the 8.30 a.m. slot earmarked for Clayton had been filled with a last-minute meeting, which I'd feel obliged to attend at the expense of my boxercise. Despite my pointing this out as gently as I could, the following week the same thing would happen, and instead of going for my soul-enriching power-walk I'd be sat around a committee room table, discussing Christmas card designs. All this started to create a palpable tension among the team. Perhaps a few of them weren't taking my requests seriously; understandably so, maybe, because I'd attempted weight-loss plans before that had come to nothing. And they, no doubt, found it frustrating to have to organise a jam-packed schedule around my morning workouts. In the end I had to put my foot down.

'Look, I know there's a crushing demand on the diary,' I said, during a pow-wow I'd convened, 'but I'm trying my best to structure a lifestyle plan, and to implement a few rules and routines. These exercise sessions are so important to me, and I really need your help.'

I added that if any more morning meetings happened to clash with my walks or workouts, I would simply not attend, full stop. Amid much rolling of eyes (I could only imagine what they were muttering under their breath) my staff took my comments on board, and agreed to protect that diary time. Indeed, once they realised the true extent of my commitment and determination, the rest of my team bought into the whole thing and offered me a great deal of support and encouragement. Health and well-being soon became a common topic of conversation in the office – somewhat ironic, since I'd avoided broaching the subject for years – and we'd readily compare and contrast our own experiences.

Sometimes, my colleagues and I would go for lunchtime walks around Westminster, walking over to the South Bank, past the London Eye, the National Theatre and the Royal Festival Hall. If it happened to be raining, we'd pace the House of Commons corridors instead.

'Who fancies a stroll?' I'd ask, especially if we'd been confined to the office all morning. 'Let's get our blood pumping, eh, and stretch our legs. Sitting still for four hours is no good for anybody.'

Later that September, the annual Labour Party conference took place at the Brighton Centre, comprising its usual mix of speeches, debates and motions, followed by convivial get-togethers and drinks receptions with members and delegates. However, compared with the previous year's gathering in Liverpool, it turned out to be an altogether different experience for me. This time, unlike 12 months previously, I neither touched a drop of alcohol, nor ate my weight in buffet food. For once, I didn't find myself hogging the karaoke machine, or joining in a drunken singalong to

'The Red Flag'. Instead, every evening I fastidiously went to bed at 9 p.m., keen to avoid these after-hours temptations and determined to stick to my regime.

'Hey, Tom, where are you going?' exclaimed a member of the Unite union, Jim Mowatt, as he spotted me in the lobby of my hotel, about to take a Waitrose chicken salad and a tub of Greek yoghurt up to my room. 'You not coming for a drink, then?'

. 'Just taking it a little bit easier this year,' I replied with a smile. 'Got an important speech tomorrow. Going to get my head down so I can wake up feeling nice and clear-headed.'

'Oh, OK...' he said, shrugging his shoulders. 'Fair enough, I s'pose. But you know where we are if you change your mind.'

I could totally understand his bewilderment. He had attended conferences with me for 25 years, and had never once known me to decline the offer of grub and Guinness.

Not only was I going to bed early to get my beauty sleep, I was also getting up at 5.30 a.m. to achieve my latest 10,000-step target. In fact, if any colleagues or comrades expressed the desire to talk politics with me during the conference, I told them I'd only agree to a chat if they accompanied me on one of my five-mile walks along the coastline. I remember strolling from Brighton to Hove with my good mate James Gurling (a lifelong Liberal Democrat, who was attending our conference in his corporate communications role), taking in the lovely sea views and marvelling at the magnificent beachside mansions. James couldn't quite get his head around my newfound lifestyle change – he'd known me as Tommy Two-Dinners for years – and, after we'd returned to the hotel, he reluctantly admitted that he'd found it difficult to keep up with my walking pace.

'Have to say, I'm bloody impressed,' he said. 'Fair play to you, mate.'

'This is just the beginning, my friend,' I replied.

My deputy leader's speech took place on the penultimate evening, and was a rallying cry for all delegates to maintain pressure on the flagging Conservative Party.

'Yes, there's hard work to do and no, we mustn't be complacent,' I said, 'but Jeremy Corbyn has broken the spell of fear the Tories sought to cast on this country. He has helped us all to remember that politics should be about inspiring hope, not peddling despair. He has shown us again what a real alternative to Toryism looks like and what it can achieve.'

It went down pretty well, I think, although the next day's *Guardian* cartoon, sketched by the inimitable Steve Bell, ruthlessly lampooned me.

'Brighton Fatberg Spotted,' ran the caption, above a huge caricature of yours truly looming over the comparatively svelte figure of our party leader.

Fatberg? Ha! Not for long… I thought, before wondering whether Bell would have used similar fat-shaming terminology had he parodied a female Member of Parliament. Being an overweight male MP seemed to justify such satire and, despite it being a grotesque portrayal, I was expected to laugh along and suck it up.

On the final day of the conference, as soon as Jeremy Corbyn's speech finished, I headed straight out of the Brighton Centre and hailed a cab to Gatwick Airport. Five hours later I was enjoying a meal in a Torremolinos restaurant, La Taberna de Guaro, talking diet and nutrition with a well-known TV weather presenter, as you do. Her advice, as it happened, would change my life.

I first met Clare Nasir, who came to national prominence while working for GMTV, through mutual friends. She and her husband, BBC 6 Music DJ Chris Hawkins, were good pals with fellow Labour MP Gloria De Piero, who happened to be married to James Robinson, my former communications director.

Gloria and I had known each other for years, and during our twenties had even shared an apartment together in London. I was by no means the perfect flatmate, as my friend will attest. Once, following a boozy night out, I returned home and put some boil-in-the-bag kippers on the hob for an early-hours snack. I then staggered into the lounge and promptly fell asleep on the sofa. The water evaporated, the plastic melted and soon the flat was filled with acrid smoke and the aroma of burnt fish.

'Are you trying to bloody kill us, Tom?' I vaguely remember Gloria yelling as she ran into the kitchen in her pyjamas, flinging the pan into the sink and flapping at the plumes of smoke. It took weeks, and countless air fresheners, for us to get rid of the smell.

Our friendship continued regardless, and in September 2017 Gloria, James and I decided to go abroad for a few days during the parliamentary break. An autumn recess was always scheduled to accommodate the various party conferences, and a cheap week on the Costa del Sol seemed just the ticket. Clare and Chris happened to be there at the same time, and we all decided to meet up one night. Clare and I chatted for ages in the restaurant. Like me, she'd once experienced her own weight struggles and, by completely overhauling her diet and fitness regime, she had since undergone a total lifestyle transformation.

Coming from a scientific background – she was a trained meteorologist – Clare had conducted meticulous research into various nutrition programmes, reading widely and furnishing herself with as much information as possible. In the end, she chose not to proceed down the conventional low-fat, low-calorie Eatwell Plate-style route. She instead embraced the low-carb, high-fat (LCHF) philosophy of so-called 'ketogenic' nutrition, a concept that I'd come across as I'd ploughed through my extensive reading list. I was intrigued to learn more about it – Clare had lost so much weight, and looked a picture of health and vitality – and, over a couple of glasses of Rioja, she gave me the rundown.

Ketogenic nutrition, I discovered, was a regime that drastically reduced the carbohydrate in your diet and replaced it with fat and non-industrially-produced oils (it had originated in the 1920s, having been prescribed for children with drug-resistant epilepsy). This reduction in carbohydrate meant that your body effectively 'learned' how to reach a metabolic state called ketosis, which then enabled your body to draw down on fat stores to produce energy by turning fat into acids in the liver, known as ketones. The Western diet very often ensured that the body only ever used glucose to provide energy, yet by restricting carbs through fasting or diet, ketogenic nutrition allowed the body to become 'fat-adapted' in order to provide fat-burning as a fuel source. Many who followed the nutritional programme claimed that it reduced sugar cravings and feelings of hunger.

Clare's LCHF keto diet predominantly comprised meat, poultry, fish, dairy products, oils and vegetables. All manner of starchy carbohydrates (pasta, rice, grains and potatoes, for example) were strictly forbidden, as were sugary carbs in all their many guises. Highly processed convenience foods were wiped off the menu, too, in favour of natural, wholesome, home-cooked alternatives.

Typical keto-friendly meals could consist of bacon and eggs for breakfast – with no toast, of course – and a chicken, avocado and leafy green salad for lunch. Dinner might be a rib-eye steak with broccoli and cauliflower, followed by fresh raspberries and double cream for dessert. Snacks and nibbles could include a handful of nuts or a couple of chunks of dark chocolate (although the latter had to be a variety with 80 per cent cocoa solids, to ensure the sugar content was low). Due to its carb content, beer was a no-no, but the occasional glass of wine, or a measure of vodka, was permitted. Eating out 'keto-style' was eminently doable, it seemed, by adapting certain restaurant dishes – forgoing the mashed potato with the pork chops, for example, and ordering spinach instead – and by avoiding others that weren't suitable.

'Have to say, Clare, I really like the sound of that.'

'Well, all I can say is that it works for me,' she replied. 'I love the meals, and like the fact that they're so filling. I never have any hunger pangs.'

I then explained to Clare how things currently stood with me: how, since the summer, I'd commenced a fitness programme, and how I'd started to monitor and reduce my sugary snacks and starchy carbs in an attempt to lose weight and control my insulin levels.

'I'm pleased with the way my fitness is going,' I said, 'but I know I won't lose weight with exercise alone. I need to really drill down into my diet and nutrition. I think it needs more structure and refinement.'

Like her, I'd done plenty of research – much of which had pointed me in the direction of LCHF programmes – but I'd not really found the impetus to go the whole hog.

'Maybe now's the time for you to move up a gear,' said Clare with a smile, adding that not only could ketogenic nutrition help me shed some weight, but that it might also help to manage my type 2 diabetes. She promised to send me some useful links to keto-related websites and podcasts, too, that had helped her on her way.

For the next few days I couldn't get our conversation out

of my head. I spent a good deal of the holiday sitting under a parasol, glued to my tablet, watching the YouTube channels and listening to the podcasts that Clare had recommended. The more I gleaned, and the more I learned, the more convinced I became that this nutritional credo was right for me. Once I returned to the UK, I vowed, I would put my own ketogenic plan into action, and I would do my utmost to stick to it.

The prospect of this was so exciting that it quite literally put a spring in my step. Toward the end of my week in Torremolinos, and for the first time in decades, I went for a jog. It may have been from one palm tree to another – and it may have left me sweating cobs in the searing Spanish sun – but, to me, it represented yet another important milestone.

CHAPTER FOUR

Downsizing

With Clare Nasir's advice still ringing in my ears, I flew back to the UK keener than ever to delve deep into the world of low-carb, high-fat nutrition. I needed to understand, as best as I could, whether this rather strict and prescriptive regime would work for me, whether it was right for my body and whether it could take Project Weight Loss to a whole new level. I was as busy as ever with work, both at Westminster and in my constituency, but whenever I had a spare half-hour I'd pick up a book or download a podcast, absorbing as much detail and information as I could.

The Diet Doctor website, to which I subscribed on Clare's recommendation, was a particularly key resource. Established in 2007, and originating from Sweden, it provided a platform for a group of clinicians who were keen to question and challenge public health advice regarding many aspects of nutrition. It gave me access to a raft of scientific research papers and video content, including studies and lectures by the brilliant Dr Jason Fung, a Canadian nephrologist with a special interest in diabetes and obesity who had treated thousands of patients. Dr Fung avidly promoted intermittent fasting as a method of losing weight. He believed that this was a way of tackling the underlying causes of many metabolic syndrome conditions linked to hyperinsulinaemia (whereby there was too much insulin in the blood relative to the level of glucose). He suggested that patients fasted for 24 hours, two or three times a week, or for 16 hours, five to six times per week, preferably having previously sought the advice of a physician.

'Fasting is the simplest and surest method to force your body to burn sugar,' he wrote in his acclaimed book, *The Diabetes Code.*

> Fasting is merely the flip side of eating: if you are not eating, you are fasting. When you eat, your body stores food energy; when you fast, your body burns food energy. And glucose is the most easily accessible source of food energy. Therefore, if you lengthen your periods of fasting, you can burn off the stored sugar. While it may sound severe, fasting is literally the oldest dietary therapy known and has been practiced throughout human history without problems.

I was also nudged in the direction of Jeff Volek and Stephen Phinney, a pair of academics based at the University of Ohio whose seminal work, *The Art and Science of Low Carbohydrate Living*, I read from cover to cover. A highly technical publication aimed primarily at health professionals, it promised, by publishing the authors' various findings and experiments, to explain how a low-carbohydrate diet could be suitable for long-term use. While it wasn't the easiest of reads for a non-medic like myself, I was still able to extrapolate that, through diet, the human body could be changed at a cellular biology level. Importantly, the authors strongly suggested that general nutrition advice, as represented by the Eatwell Plate, was no longer fit for purpose. Instead, practitioners needed to relate such guidance to an individual's unique physiology.

What the book did, fundamentally, was reaffirm that there was a different, nonconformist pathway toward weight loss.

'Seems you're on your own, Tom,' I remember thinking to myself, as it looked more likely than ever that I'd be contravening those official dietary guidelines.

Dr Phinney also acted as a medical advisor for an organisation in the US, Virta Health. This commercial outfit helped to treat people with type 2 diabetes by putting them on a ketogenic diet, and by offering them advice and support. Virta Health's research, which I read with interest, revealed a remarkable rate of T2D reversal among their patients, and suggested that ketogenic nutrition was indeed the crucial factor.

During my Kennington Park power-walks (which, if I felt sprightly, occasionally broke into jogs), I liked to listen to the illuminating *2 Keto Dudes* podcast. It featured a pair of middle-aged men, Richard Morris and Carl Franklin – from Australia and the United States respectively – who had become something of a podcasting phenomenon. Over the years, both had suffered with obesity-related health issues and metabolic syndrome disorders, and both had questioned the health and nutrition advice dished out by health authorities in their native countries. Separately, they'd embarked upon a ketogenic nutrition regime – the results had been remarkable, with regard to their weight loss and their general well-being – and, along their journeys, the two men's paths had crossed on various social networks.

Realising that they had a great deal in common, Morris and Franklin decided to join forces and set up their own podcast, its premise being to extol the virtues of their ketogenic lifestyle (a 'hardcore version of the low-carb diet', they called it) by outlining personal experiences and by offering pertinent advice. One week the chosen topic could be 'Keto for Absolute Beginners', and the following week it could be 'Eating Fat to Satiety'. As well as sharing keto diet and recipe tips (they had an infectious passion for food) they also conducted fascinating interviews with an impressive array of scientists and clinicians, many of whom were swimming against the tide of standard nutritional guidelines. Biochemist Ivor Cummins and Harvard professor David Ludwig made a big impression on me when they discussed heart science and ketogenic research respectively, as did Peter Brukner, an author and sports medicine physician, who led an anti-sugar campaign in Australia.

My podcast obsession led to the serendipitous discovery of other so-named 'biohackers'. This fairly modern concept saw scientifically minded individuals choosing to fine-tune their own environment, or their own body, in order to improve their health and upgrade their day-to-day living. One such exponent was a Silicon Valley entrepreneur by the name of Dave Asprey. During his thirties, Asprey's general health had taken a nosedive – he'd become clinically obese, with a litany of ailments that included chronic fatigue – and, since other diets had failed him, he'd researched and developed his own self-styled 'Bulletproof Diet'. High in fat, medium in protein and low in carbohydrate, it focused upon quality rather than quantity (Asprey acquired his fat from avocado, butter and coconut oil, for example, and only ate meat from animals that had been grass-fed) and it aimed to trigger weight loss through ketosis.

In 2014, having already lost nearly 100lb (45 kilos) on the diet, he decided to outline his credo in a book, *The Bulletproof Diet*, which led to an associated podcast, website and YouTube channel. It was his somewhat unconventional take on a hot beverage that really put him on the map, however. I remember listening to one of his podcasts in bed one night, utterly enthralled as this charismatic Californian outlined the 'Bulletproof Coffee' backstory. In 2004, during a mountain trek in Tibet, Asprey had found himself ascending to 18,000 feet above sea level and experiencing temperatures of -10°F. Battling severe fatigue and exhaustion, and feeling his energy levels tumbling, he'd staggered into a nearby travellers' hut for shelter and sustenance. A friendly local had handed him what he described as 'a creamy cup of yak's butter tea', which, by all accounts, was the staple drink for those who lived in this harsh, high-altitude environment. It proved to have an amazing effect upon him.

'The drink instantly rejuvenated me,' reflected Dave. 'It was like a switch was flipped on in my brain and body.'

He was intrigued as to why this concoction had such a positive effect – he'd felt invigorated, mentally and physically – and, as a result, he spent some time researching the restorative properties of yak's butter (a fairly niche concept, let's be honest). He then developed his own West Coast version, using fresh coffee beans instead of tea and substituting the Tibetan butter with grass-fed cows' butter. For extra zing he then added some of his trademarked Brain Octane Oil into the mix – derived from coconut palm oil, it claimed to amplify energy and aid cognition – and Bulletproof Coffee was born. It soon caught on in California, and became something of a phenomenon in other Western countries.

It all sounds a bit new-agey, I remember thinking, *but if the science is sound, I must give it a go one day...*

Dave Asprey's *Bulletproof Radio* podcasts were a turning point for me. I didn't agree with everything his special guests said, but these interviews exposed me to people on the frontline of research, pioneers in their field, who were testing this very embryonic idea of effecting biological control upon the human body. I also identified with Dave's nerdy, obsessional tendencies, and I couldn't help but be inspired by the way he'd revolutionised his whole life through nutrition. He was, for me, a game-changer.

My own attempt at biohacking (albeit entry-level) got under way in the first week of October, when I decided to fully embrace a ketogenic diet. From then on, I'd restrict starchy carbohydrates to no more than 5 per cent of my daily intake, sticking to around 20g per day. I would opt instead for protein-rich foods — so plenty of red meat, poultry, fish and dairy — in addition to low-sugar fruits and vegetables like blueberries and broccoli. In order to combat the pangs and cravings that came with sugar withdrawal, and to stop myself feeling hungry, I'd increase the amount of saturated fat in my diet (including butter, cheese and double cream). Alcohol would be strictly limited to the occasional glass of dry white wine or a vodka and soda.

I remember sitting down and formulating a meal plan for the week (much of the recipes having been cribbed from 2 Keto Dudes) before heading off to Tesco with an extra-long shopping list. Into the trolley went lamb chops, salmon steaks, chicken thighs, leafy greens and mixed salad for my main dishes. Then, for desserts, I grabbed punnets of blackberries and raspberries (both had lower fructose levels compared with other fruit) as well as tubs of full-fat Greek yoghurt and double cream. For snacking, I stocked up on my favourite hard and soft cheeses, and threw in a few large bags of unsalted walnuts and macadamia nuts.

I blanked out any thoughts of sugary snacks, fizzy drinks and processed food, bypassing the aisles that would've usually been my first port of call, and ignoring the empty calories that used to form the basis of my former diet. Indeed, for the first time in ages I genuinely enjoyed doing the 'big shop'. I had always seen it as a time-sapping chore, a mere trolley-dash, but this time around I found myself scrutinising labels and squeezing produce instead of mindlessly plucking the same old items from oft-visited shelves.

Admittedly, my total spend at the till was marginally more expensive than normal, but I reckoned that my new keto regime would save me money in the long term. By ditching sugary snacks and junk food, and by cooking from scratch at home instead of relying on convenience meals (many of which went to waste), I was pretty sure that, in real terms, I'd be able to reduce my monthly outlay.

I logged the first day on my ketogenic-style diet on Monday 9 October 2017. For breakfast, I ate a two-egg omelette, with two rashers of fried bacon cooked in butter on a low heat. Lunch comprised scrambled egg, again with two rashers of bacon (I still couldn't quite believe that two of my favourite foodstuffs were part of a 'diet'). My snack quota comprised a small handful of nuts and, when I felt a serious hunger pang, a few blackberries with double cream.

Later that day I went out for dinner with my friends, Lord Roy Kennedy and his wife, Baroness Alicia Kennedy, at the Kennington Tandoori, an eatery popular with MPs and Westminster folk and notable for its wall-to-wall photos of politicians. That particular evening I eschewed my regular order of chicken dhansak, tarka dhal and peshwari naan, instead opting for tandoori chicken and a small serving of saag paneer (a tasty dish of Indian cheese with spinach puree).

'So you're telling me that you can't even have a naan on this plan of yours?' asked Roy as he tore off a strip of bread, using it to wipe the curry sauce off his plate. 'With your appetite, how on earth are you going to cope?'

'Well, let's just see how it goes, eh?' I said, with a shrug, as a devilish voice dared me to lean over the table and grab what remained of Roy's naan. My fingers were twitching, and my resolve was wavering, but somehow I resisted the urge.

As my first day on keto came to a close, my stomach felt pleasantly full. I hadn't suffered any energy slumps – so no falling asleep on the sofa once I'd returned from the restaurant – and had genuinely enjoyed the food I'd eaten. The MyFitnessPal log showed that I'd consumed a total of 2,330 calories, with a macronutrient breakdown of 5 per cent carbohydrates, 72 per cent fat and 23 per cent protein. Even though I'd kept those carbs nice and low, the macro balance was pretty challenging for me to look at, since it seriously contradicted the government's Eatwell guidelines.

A whole week went by, and not once did I deviate from my plan. I spent much more time cooking for myself at home, and preparing my own packed lunches, although the number of serviceable recipe books had diminished. Many of the Italian-themed titles had to be given away – the prevalence of pasta, pizza and risotto severely limited my options – and the same applied to all my rice-and-noodle-heavy Chinese cookbooks. I instead turned to online recipes for ideas and inspiration (notably the 2 Keto Dudes' menu planners) and also bought a copy of the wonderful *Ginger Pig Meat Book*, by Tim Wilson and Fran Warde. With these resources to hand, I was able to prepare an appetising repertoire of meals from scratch that included crispy pork belly with pork scratchings and steamed runner beans; fried halloumi cheese with avocado and buttered spinach; pan-fried salmon with broccoli and cauliflower and slow-roast chilli beef with a leafy green salad.

On days four, five and six I did experience some cravings, however – I surmised it was my body demanding a sugar fix – yet I always managed, somehow, to quell the hunger pangs by gulping down a big dollop of thick double cream. I would be lying, though, if I said this felt like a normal thing to do. Despite my being well-versed in ketogenic nutrition, and its core principles of satiation through fat, the act of glugging double cream to relieve my appetite just seemed, well… a little weird. Part of me still needed convincing that this was actually going to work.

Keep the faith, Tom, I said to myself. *Believe in the science, and see it through…*

Around the same time, I also suffered mild symptoms of what is commonly termed 'keto flu', characterised by a certain feverishness, grogginess and tiredness in the wake of serious sugar and carb withdrawal. It was short-lived, thankfully, and by the beginning of Keto Week Two I was waking up feeling absolutely bloody brilliant. It was remarkable, really. The general malaise that used to greet me when my alarm went off – aching joints, sore back, banging head, breathlessness – simply disappeared, and I instead sprang out of my bed feeling so much brighter, sharper and happier. My quality of sleep improved massively (I didn't have to make any early-hours trips to the loo; previously it had been two pees per night) and my digestive system seemed much better, with my increased vegetable intake 'keeping me regular', as they say.

And, more to the point, I wasn't hungry any more. No pangs, no cravings, no rumbling stomach. I could barely believe this was happening to me.

With the rest of my eating programme going swimmingly, the time soon came to give Dave Asprey's Bulletproof Coffee a whirl. I was keen to decide for myself whether this newfangled hot drink was a hipster fad or a restorative elixir, and used the Bulletproof website as my guide.

1) Firstly, I brewed enough coffee for one cup, using freshly ground beans (I bought some Monmouth Coffee, the espresso blend; I thought I'd treat myself to some quality stuff, seeing as I was denying myself alcohol).
2) Then, I allowed it to cool for a minute or so (being destined for the liquidiser, it couldn't be boiling hot).
3) I added one teaspoon of Ketosource MCT oil, which I bought online (it's pretty potent stuff, so I started with one teaspoon per cup, and worked my way up to one to two tablespoons over several days).
4) Into the mix went two tablespoons of unsalted butter (grass-fed is best, according to Dave). I remember chuckling to myself and thinking *I can't believe I'm doing this* as I stirred it in.
5) I poured the mixture into a blender and pulsed it for thirty seconds, until it looked foamy…
6) …and then I drank it.

I was, as it happened, pleasantly surprised. The drink was more than palatable and tasted remarkably creamy, like a caffè latte, and didn't have the greasy aftertaste that I'd expected. The first few days on Bulletproof Coffee didn't have a discernible effect upon me, though, and there came a point when I wondered whether I'd actually experience the clarity and vitality that had so transformed Dave Asprey. However, within a week or two I certainly began to feel the benefit. With this turbocharged coffee coursing through my system – in tandem with my fresh new diet plan and my blossoming exercise regime – I felt pumped up with energy, both mentally and physically. It was as though I had more petrol in the tank. At work, for instance, whenever I trawled through reports and briefings, I seemed better able to absorb data and information. If I held committee meetings in parliament, or delivered speeches at conferences, I felt somehow more articulate and quick-witted.

Back at home – especially when I had my son and daughter in tow – I felt increasingly alert and attentive. More than ever before, I found myself talking with the children about music and sport, and what they'd done at school, and I was no longer falling asleep during our bedtime storytelling. There were fewer distracted thoughts buzzing around my head – my concentration span had lengthened – and there was less twitchiness to reach for my mobile or my laptop. Indeed, for years Saoirse had mimicked my constant phone use (whenever I was deep in conversation, she'd extend her thumb and little finger, holding them to her ear) but she soon noticed the difference in my behaviour.

'Daddy, thank you for not being on the phone so much any more,' she announced one day, completely blindsiding me and causing my bottom lip to wobble. This newfound lucidity made me realise just how bleary and foggy-headed I must have been in my kids' company. It also made me regret that, for their sake, I'd not implemented these lifestyle changes sooner.

Bulletproof Coffee promptly became an integral part of my early-morning routine, two or three times a week. I would get out of bed, head to the bathroom, step on the scales, log my measurements, go downstairs, grind the coffee, put the pot on the stove, add the butter and MCT oil, let it percolate for five minutes, have a shower in the meantime and then return to the kitchen to crank up the blender. I enjoyed the ritualistic, almost ceremonial element; it helped me reinforce the idea that I was embedding positive habits, and that I was diligently reorganising my life. It helped me to practise a certain mindfulness, too; the mere act of making this enriching cup of coffee gave me a sense of being 'in the moment', and allowed me to feel that I was doing something purposeful to aid my well-being.

Sometimes, if I was too time-pressured to prepare a cooked breakfast, or if I was seeing Clayton for an early-morning workout, I'd fix myself one of my special coffees instead. For me, it was a more than adequate substitution; its high saturated fat content suppressed my hunger for hours, enabling me to remain full until lunchtime, and allowing me to resist the temptation of a mid-morning snack.

'Chocolate Hobnob, Tom?' I'd be asked during a meeting

in a Commons committee room, as the refreshments trolley was trundled in.

'No thank you, I'm fine,' I'd say, smiling, reaching for the water jug to top up my glass.

It had taken a long time, but I'd finally found myself in full control of my thoughts and actions, and possessing the inner strength to avoid a Cookie Monster-style biscuit binge. Shunning that chocolate Hobnob, without a single pang of regret, was a truly amazing feeling.

Although I believed wholeheartedly in the Bulletproof, some of my loved ones reckoned I'd completely lost the plot. Whenever I extolled its virtues, and related Dave Asprey's story (Tibetan yak's milk and all), I was met with derisive snorts and raised eyebrows.

'Butter in coffee? Ugh, that sounds vile,' said my friend Fraser Kemp as we chatted on the phone one evening, during which call I'd tried to explain how, thanks to a combination of Bulletproof, keto and exercise, I was feeling so much better in mind and body. The next time Fraser and I met, however, he probably detected a certain vivacity in me that he perhaps hadn't seen for decades, and the initial cynicism appeared to melt away.

'So, tell me again, Tom, exactly how much butter do you put in that coffee?' he asked. 'And can I use margarine instead?'

'Sorry mate,' I said, grinning, 'margarine is on the banned list.'

*

While my low-carb, high-fat eating plan had taken early inspiration from the work of Dr Michael Mosley and Professor Roy Taylor (and, more latterly, my friend Clare Nasir and the 2 Keto Dudes), I continued to encounter other books and studies that crystallised my way of thinking. *The Pioppi Diet*, co-written by cardiologist Dr Aseem Malhotra and documentary-maker Donal O'Neill, was one such example. It took its inspiration from a tiny village in southern Italy whose inhabitants enjoyed a longer than usual life expectancy; their Mediterranean-style diet was found to be low in sugar, starchy carbohydrates and processed foods, which, according to the book, probably helped reduce their risk of developing chronic conditions such as heart disease and type 2 diabetes.

Like me, *The Pioppi Diet*'s authors viewed the nutritional advice meted out by the UK government since the 1980s as flawed and outdated, especially its demonisation of saturated fat and the glorification of calorie-controlled diets.

'Be prepared for everything you know and believe to be true to be turned on its head,' the book's introduction stated. 'Misguided public health messages and the marketing campaigns that push them continue to mislead doctors, the public and politicians, but it's time for that to change...'

It was the authors' holistic credo that particularly appealed to my sensibilities. While an LCHF diet remained at the core of their programme (its recipes and meal plans were excellent), the book advocated an all-embracing, big-picture approach to well-being and weight loss. Those with aspirations of a long and healthy life needed to learn how to manage their stress levels, it was suggested, and needed to optimise their sleep patterns and maintain meaningful social interaction. Exercise and activity – or 'mindful movement' – had to be at the forefront, too, in order to avoid the myriad health problems associated with a sedentary lifestyle. This didn't necessarily mean pumping weights or pounding treadmills (after all, there were no gyms in the village of Pioppi) but could instead comprise a brisk 30-minute walk or a regular series of stretches.

The Pioppi Diet deepened my interest in the idea of survival and longevity, and provided me with some thought-provoking theory and guidance. It felt good to contemplate how long I was going to live, not how soon I was going to die.

On a more practical and culinary level, the book helped me to understand that I needed to eat real food, not processed food, and also widened my repertoire of tasty low-carb recipes. I remember whipping up pork chops with sage butter for myself one evening, and as I carefully chewed each mouthful, savouring the meat-and-herb flavour combination, I suddenly realised that my sense of taste had definitely intensified since I'd quit junk food. My taste buds had been dulled by three decades of bland 'n' beige stodge, and were gradually acclimatising themselves to decent, wholesome fare.

This is so flippin' good, I thought to myself. *Beats a stuffed-crust Meat Feast any day of the week.*

Although I was becoming quite au fait with home cooking, I still enjoyed the occasional meal out with friends or family. Dining in restaurants, keto-style, was pretty easy in larger cities. At Yo! Sushi, in Manchester's Piccadilly station, I would choose tuna sashimi (which doesn't have rice), rather than sushi, and at the Covent Garden branch of Five Guys I would plump for a large beef patty with cheese. The staff there were happy to serve it wrapped up in an iceberg lettuce leaf so that I could eat it like a regular burger and, as I tucked in to my bespoke, keto-style meal I remember thinking how my younger, gluttonous self would have pissed himself laughing at the very sight of it.

As for desserts, I avoided all manner of cakes and pastries, either opting for fresh berries with cream or a cheeseboard with grapes (minus any sugary chutney or carb-laden crackers, of course). I ended up becoming a bit of a cheese connoisseur, in fact, using my revitalised taste buds to differentiate between a wedge of Wensleydale and a chunk of Caerphilly.

Adhering to my eating regime was slightly trickier in West Bromwich – there wasn't the same breadth of choice – but there were ways to get around it, and there were venues that were more keto-friendly than others. I had been a long-time patron of the Vine on Roebuck Street, one of the many 'Desi' pubs that had sprung up in the area, renowned for serving top Punjabi fare in great British boozers. Its grill room was legendary, and in bygone times I'd often capped off a beer-fuelled Saturday night with a large plateful of methi chicken and rice, mopping up the delicious Punjabi 'gravy' with hunks of freshly baked naan bread.

When I paid a visit, post-keto, I ditched the naan and the gravy, though, and requested two portions of methi chicken, but minus the rice. The Vine's proprietor, a lovely guy called Suki, looked flummoxed.

'You sure that's going to be enough for you, Tom?' he asked. 'No gravy? No naan? No rice? Are you not feeling well tonight?'

'I'm good, Suki, just fancy something different,' I replied, smiling to myself as he looked at me with deep concern. 'But don't scrimp on that chicken, eh?'

While eating out in restaurants was relatively straightforward on a keto diet, eating on the hop during the working day could be difficult. I tried to cobble together my own packed lunches if I was on my travels but, on the occasions when this wasn't possible, I'd often struggle to find keto-friendly options. On the train, I'd regularly find myself having to peel roast chicken slices off a sandwich roll – fresh salads were few and far between – and sometimes I'd have to resort to munching on a few bags of mixed nuts. In a certain high-street coffee emporium, often found in airports and railway stations, there was virtually nothing I could grab from the glass display cabinets, save a bowl of fruit salad (and even then I'd have to take out the high-carb banana and mango). No doubt some of my travelling companions saw my actions as rather extreme, and very pernickety ('surely ONE chocolate muffin isn't going to kill you, Tom?') but I was determined that nothing was going to throw me off course.

Within days of starting keto, in that second week of October, my weight had begun to plummet. When I'd stepped on the scales in early August, at the beginning of the summer recess, the needle had rested at 308lb (22 stone or 140 kilos). By the end of September – having commenced some gentle exercise, and having started a gradual reduction of carbs and sugar – I'd come in at 289lb (131 kilos) and, on Monday 9 October (the day I returned from Torremolinos), I'd weighed a total of 281.8lb (128 kilos). I had shed nearly two stone, or 13 kilos, in two months (amazing, really, since I'd only made moderate tweaks to my diet) but I still found myself in the XXXL size range, still with a high body mass index, and still clinically obese.

It was only when I applied strict ketogenic nutrition principles – ultra-low carbs, and comparatively high fats – that I began to see remarkable results. During that very first week, I inputted the following data into my MyFitnessPal app:

Monday 9 October: 281.8lb
Tuesday 10 October: 279.1lb
Wednesday 11 October: 278.9lb
Thursday 12 October: 276.2lb
Friday 13 October: 277.4lb (a slight increase here,
which can happen for a variety of reasons. Perhaps I had
some water retention that day)
Saturday 14 October: 274.6lb
Sunday 15 October: 274.8lb

After just one week of keto, I'd lost seven pounds, half a stone (three kilos). *One* week. *Seven* pounds. I was totally and utterly elated. This may sound a little melodramatic but, apart from the birth of my kids, it was the best week of my life. Finally — *finally* — my own deeds and actions had benefited my body, not failed it, and I'd actually made a difference. And, not only had I lost half a stone, I'd done so without any sense of food deprivation, and by eating a succession of fabulous meals. From smashed avocado and bacon in the morning, to barbecue ribs and salad in the evening, not once had I felt remotely peckish.

I had to speak to someone about it, to shout about my good news, so I told my pal David Wild after we'd finished walking around Kennington Park.

'You'll never guess what's happened,' I said, breathlessly reeling off all the MyFitnessPal stats. I must have sounded like a total nerd, but I felt too exhilarated to care.

'Bloody well done, mate, losing half a stone in a week is amazing,' he said.

'I feel marvellous,' I replied, thrilled that I'd successfully embedded an eating plan that seemed to perfectly suit my needs. 'Fifty-one years old, David, and I'm finally starting to take care of myself.'

As my keto regime gathered pace, and my life became more disciplined, I got into the habit of measuring myself more regularly, from my glucose levels to my blood pressure. Only by closely monitoring my own data could I properly chart my progress, I reckoned, and I would carefully pencil all the relevant data into a little notebook. By my own admission, in the past I'd been negligent in this respect, especially in the wake of my T2D diagnosis. For instance, I'd never performed a blood glucose finger-prick test before (even though I'd been given the kit), although that was probably down to a combination of fear, denial and laziness.

Every morning I assiduously measured my fasting blood sugars and on alternate days I checked my blood pressure. High blood pressure, or hypertension, was very common in my family, and even though I was taking medication it remained a concern. Deep down I knew that much of it was related to weight, but over the years I'd conveniently convinced myself that it was genetic, and that there was nothing I could do about it. Examining the daily data was a sobering experience – I had stage two hypertension, which was classed as severely high blood pressure – but it also helped me to focus. Each daily reading may have made my heart sink, but it also motivated me to put on my trainers and get moving.

I also began to monitor my ketone levels on a daily basis. This was to ascertain whether I'd entered that Holy Grail-like state of ketosis, whereby my body was drawing down its energy source from fat stores rather than carbohydrate stores. This again involved using a finger-prick with a test strip that, when measured against a blood ketone index, revealed my ketone count. This, combined with my blood glucose reading, provided me with a ratio – the glucose-ketone index (GKI) – which indicated whether or not I was at the right level of ketosis to promote fat-burning, to reduce obesity and to tackle insulin resistance. Getting a handle on ketosis was important in terms of Project Weight Loss, since it allowed me to establish whether I was ingesting the right balance of foodstuffs. It also helped me to understand how my body was responding, both nutritionally and biologically, to this whole new way of eating.

I spent Christmas with Siobhan and the kids at her parents' home in Yorkshire. I lapsed a little bit, diet-wise – after three 'dry' months, I couldn't resist a few celebratory glasses of white wine – but I still managed to keep the dinner itself pretty keto-friendly. My in-laws, Paul and Karen, were magnificent cooks and served me up a delicious plate of roast turkey, Brussels sprouts, baby carrots, red cabbage and cauliflower cheese. The previous year I'd helped to prepare some speciality 'trimmings' (namely Tom Kerridge's glazed carrots and Delia Smith's red cabbage) but, since both contained copious amounts of sugar, on this occasion my considerate in-laws had made some plainer versions. I politely swerved the roast potatoes and cranberry sauce, though – not easy, since the extra-crispy spuds looked superb – and for dessert I opted for the festive cheeseboard instead of the Christmas pudding and brandy sauce.

'Dad, I can't believe you're not eating this,' said Malachy, tucking into his fruit pud with gusto.

'Don't worry about me, son,' I said, smiling. 'This vintage Stilton's a winner.'

The Watson family enjoyed New Year's Eve together, too, the plan being for all four of us to attend the House of Commons firework display, an annual event attended by

MPs and support staff that raised funds for various charities. We spent the preceding afternoon trailing up and down London's Oxford Street, however, since my 12-year-old son had suddenly become fashion-conscious, and was desperate to spend his Christmas money in the sales.

While Malachy and Saoirse browsed the rails in Gap, Siobhan dragged me into Zara, suggesting that I needed to update my wardrobe since my clothes were becoming baggier by the day. I had never once crossed the threshold of this particular store; I'd always thought it looked far too trendy for me, and had assumed that my 22-stone frame would have barely fitted into the changing cubicle, let alone a pair of their trousers. Other than good ol' Marks & Spencer, I'd rarely shopped on the high street, and had instead routinely ordered clothes online from 'plus-size' retailers.

'Here you are, Tom, this is nice,' Siobhan said, holding up a blue patterned shirt, probably a tad brighter than I'd have usually worn. 'Why don't you try it on? You could wear it tonight.'

I scrutinised the label: XL. It had been a decade or so since I'd squeezed myself into that size.

'Okay...' I replied, nervously. 'Let's give it a go.'

Five minutes later I emerged from the changing room, my broad grin speaking volumes.

'It's ever-so-slightly tight-ish, but it fits,' I told Siobhan, 'and it actually looks OK.'

'Brilliant,' she said, smiling. 'I tell you what, Tom, let me treat you to this. Your first non-M&S shirt for thirty years.'

It was a very kind gesture from my former partner. This size drop was a special moment for me, and she knew it.

Malachy and Saoirse, on the other hand, spent the rest of the shopping trip affectionately ribbing me, trying (and failing) to persuade me to try on various wild and wacky designer outfits in Selfridges, now that I could finally fit into an XL. Beneath all the jesting, however, I sensed they were delighted to witness the positive change in their dad, in both attitude and appearance. I had always been a weighty, wheezing presence in their lives, but now that I was feeling better and getting fitter, I think they were really noticing the difference. That particular day I'd walked along Oxford Street without having to cling onto a wall to get my breath, for instance, and had passed by McDonald's without the urge to stop for a quarter-pounder. I hadn't lost focus mid-conversation, and I hadn't become drowsy mid-afternoon.

My newfound vigour was allowing me to engage more meaningfully with my children, and this made me feel inordinately happy. After all, my desire to get well, and to get healthy, had always been as much about Malachy and Saoirse as it had been about me. The desire to make up for lost time ran so deeply, and I wanted to be a presence in their lives for many years to come.

Later that evening, clad in our new gear, the Watson clan joined the throng on the floodlit House of Commons terrace. Greeting us were a number of friends and colleagues, including Bradford South MP Judith Cummins and Baroness Alicia Kennedy.

'Scrubbing up well, you lot,' said Alicia, smiling, eyeing

the faux-leather coat that I'd grabbed for half-price in Zara. 'Snazzy jacket, Tom.'

'Thanks very much,' I said, part of me wanting to yell 'Yeah, and guess what… it's only an EXTRA LARGE!'

As Big Ben's chimes rang out, the fireworks display kicked off. With Malachy and Saoirse by my side, I watched as a succession of rockets erupted in the night sky, their gold and silver sparkles reflected in the River Thames below. As the strains of 'Auld Lang Syne' rang out from the terrace, I found myself welling up with emotion. I'd had a great day. And I was going to have a great 2018.

CHAPTER FIVE

Healthy Turnaround

I continued to visit my GP, Dr Nazeer, albeit perhaps not with the same regularity that I'd done in the past. I was feeling so much better health-wise, and felt far more in control of my condition, and simply didn't think it necessary to be knocking on his door every two or three weeks. However, during a scheduled appointment toward the end of 2017 I'd happened to mention that I was following an ultra-low-carb ketogenic programme, that the subsequent weight loss had been dramatic and that, according to my daily fasting plasma glucose tests, my blood sugar levels had dipped to 5.7mmol/L (millimoles per litre), which, according to the chart that I'd been given, was within the 'pre-diabetic' range. He seemed pleased to find me looking brighter and lighter, albeit via unconventional methods, but was keen to manage my expectations. Technically, once the NHS tells you you're a type 2 diabetic, you're always a type 2 diabetic, and it was prudent and professional for my GP to exercise caution at this stage.

In January 2018, and following some gentle persuasion, Dr Nazeer agreed to give me an earlier-than-scheduled HbA1c blood test. This annual measurement of my long-term fasting blood sugars wasn't due for a few months but, since I was feeling so good, I wanted another in the interim. The results were astonishing. My HbA1c test came in at 4.9mmol/L, which, according to the NHS measurement guidelines, indicated that I was within the normal range (the upper end of normal, granted, but that was good enough for me). I could hardly take it in. A year ago, I'd have considered this impossible. Had I not been sitting before this very distinguished doctor I might have let slip an expletive, but I bit my tongue and said it in my head instead.

Normal. Bloody hell.

It appeared that, by controlling my own biochemistry through nutrition, I'd managed to significantly reduce my glucose levels and, for the time being, had put my type 2 diabetes into remission. Three months spent strictly monitoring my carbohydrate intake had had a transformational effect on my body, and had enabled my blood sugars to come down to within the normal range. While this was the finest personal victory I could have ever imagined, I also felt a twinge of regret. I had spent five years of my life in denial about my health issues, yet had I got my act together sooner I could have sorted it out in three months flat.

Dr Nazeer's face was a picture. For years I'd been one of his problem patients, frequently missing appointments and often mired in denial, and I'm sure he'd never imagined me making this breakthrough. Many a time I'd noticed him raising his eyebrows at me in undisguised disappointment, but on this occasion he was positively beaming. He even came over to give me a little man-hug.

'I'm so proud of you, Tom,' he said, patting me on the back. 'You really deserve this.'

'Thank you,' I replied. 'Genuinely, thank you.'

As soon as I got home I rang my brother Dan. I had been regularly updating him on my progress and he'd been hugely tolerant of his elder brother's health and exercise-related ramblings. He had also been on a weight-loss journey some years previously, and understood just how toilsome the whole process could be. Dan's lifestyle change had involved a huge amount of cycling, including a daily 20-mile pedal to work along the canal towpaths that ran from Kidderminster to West Bromwich.

'That's such great news, Tom,' he said. 'The first of many milestones, eh?'

'Let's hope so,' I replied. 'Still can't quite believe it.'

Within a few weeks, and in consultation with Dr Nazeer, I began to wean myself off metformin, my type 2 diabetes medication. From a physiological perspective, the HbA1c test (combined with my daily finger-prick test, and my improved general health) had acted as the confirmation that I was able to control my blood sugar levels through nutrition alone. From a psychological perspective, as soon as I'd realised that my diabetes was in remission, ditching the medication became my absolute goal, a symbol of success.

My weight continued on a downward trajectory, going from 252lb (114 kilos) on New Year's Day to 227lb (103 kilos) by the end of April. As the flab began to fall off, people soon cottoned on. At Westminster, fellow MPs gave me double-takes as I strode purposefully through the Commons' corridors – 'that can't be Tommy Two-Dinners,' I heard someone say – and lobby reporters began to jest in print that I was 'a political lightweight' or a 'diminished figure in Westminster'. It may not have sounded entirely flattering, but in the most literal sense it was indeed true. Some people even mistook me for a dark, slim, bespectacled colleague of mine, Karl Turner, the MP for Hull East. That amused him no end.

'Never thought I'd see the day that I'd get confused with Tom Watson,' he said, laughing.

'Time to buy yourself some different glasses,' I replied.

I also had a handful of politicians knocking on my office door, intrigued as to how I'd lost the weight. My good pal, the Labour MP for St Helens North, Conor McGinn, had not long joined the Westminster fray – in his early thirties, he was one of the younger breed of members – and had been alarmed to discover that his busy new lifestyle had led to some weight gain. I told him how a ketogenic nutrition regime had worked for me (while stressing that it wasn't the answer for everyone) and he decided to follow in my footsteps and lost a few pounds in the process.

I received a visit from a somewhat rotund backbench MP, too, whose wife had seen a photo of me in the newspapers and had insisted that he paid me a visit to discover my 'secret'.

'My other half says she won't stop bugging me until I see you,' he admitted, a little sheepishly. 'So here I am.'

'No problem at all,' I smiled. We talked for a while, and I agreed to email him my reading and research list, from Dr Michael Mosley's book to Professor Roy Taylor's study, so that he could make his own informed decision.

Three further MPs (all of whom were suffering with type 2 diabetes) decided to confide in me as well. One colleague in particular had only recently been diagnosed, and was incredibly anxious about his future health and well-being. We sat down for a private chat in my office and, as he poured his heart out, I found myself relating totally to his deep sense of fear and shame. I ended up spending a good deal of time with this MP, reassuring him that type 2 diabetes really didn't need to be a lifelong condition and explaining how, by adapting his diet and by introducing some exercise, he could even try to put it into remission.

'It's a long-term project that can have lifetime results,' I said.

'I hope you're right, Tom,' he responded. 'I'm worried as hell.'

I received support from across the political divide, too. Conservative MP Sir Nicholas Soames (grandson of Winston Churchill, no less) was a jovial individual with whom I'd always got on well, despite our ideological differences. He too had successfully slimmed down his once-bulky frame, although, unlike me, he'd followed a more conventional low-fat, low-calorie plan (he claimed to swear by yoghurt and berries for breakfast but, knowing Soames, he probably lost his weight by going down from seven courses to four). Different diets worked for different people, of course, and Nicholas had certainly found the one that best suited him.

'I can't quite believe my eyes, Tom,' he said, collaring me in the House of Commons one afternoon. 'Congratulations. What a transformation. You're a credit to parliament. You must send me your diet secrets.'

'That's very kind of you to say,' I replied. 'Much less of a squeeze on those Commons benches nowadays.'

Another Tory MP, James Duddridge, became a great support and sounding board. In the wake of a few health scares he'd lost weight and become super-fit, and along the way had developed a serious running addiction. James and I would often meet up for a light lunch in the Commons Tea Room, where we'd share our health tips, compare our experiences and try to avert our gazes from the bacon butties. Since I'd now started jogging in various parks around the capital, including St James's Park and Vauxhall Pleasure Gardens, he kept trying to tempt me into training with him, with a view to running the London Marathon. I always declined, though. Clayton the taskmaster had always stressed that the golden rule of exercise for the over-50s was DO NOT GET INJURED and I didn't want to push myself too far and hamper my progress. I appreciated the sentiment, though (the fact he'd even asked me showed me how far I'd come) but I was perfectly happy with my runs in Kennington Park.

While the majority of Westminster folk seemed very pleased for me, I occasionally found myself on the receiving end of a reverse compliment.

'Don't lose any more weight, Tom, will you?' some would say, in mildly patronising tones. 'You look fine as you are. You don't want to get too thin now, do you?'

'Let me be the judge of that,' I'd say, smiling – albeit through gritted teeth – mindful that such comments were sometimes born of envy, or suspicion. I sensed that some individuals believed that my 'new look' had some sort of ulterior motive, and was part of a cunning, premeditated bid to improve my appearance, polish my image and climb the ranks of power. This was complete and utter bollocks, of course. Nothing could have been further from the truth.

I do think, though, that some parliamentary colleagues found it hard to reconcile themselves with Tom Watson version 2.0, in particular my newfound, non-confrontational demeanour. In fact, I'd go so far as to say that some were completely infuriated by it. Once upon a time, in the midst of my sugar addiction, whenever a colleague tried to trigger me during a combative meeting I'd have bitten back with a vengeance, shouting the odds and thumping the desk like that flighty ex-union official of yesteryear.

However, post-Project Weight Loss, and positively radiating calmness and contentment, I responded to any provocation with a smile, a shrug and some softly spoken words. I could almost see the steam coming out of certain people's ears as I refused to rise to the bait.

As an MP, you expect an element of aggravation – it's par for the course to get needled by opponents, colleagues and reporters – but in my new, Zen-like state everything seemed to be washing over me. In fact, there came a point in mid-2018 when I genuinely questioned whether I was too chilled out and laid-back for the job.

My own office staff detected a change in attitude, too. According to Jo, Sarah and the team, once I quelled my sugar addiction (and cleared my brain fog) I turned into a completely different boss. I became a lot more focused in meetings, they reckoned, I could recall facts and figures without prompting, and I was much better prepared for speeches and interviews. Their jobs had become considerably easier as a result, which was good to hear, but I couldn't help but feel a little remorseful all the same.

'It must have been a nightmare for you guys at times,' I told them one afternoon, casting my mind back to those dark, dysfunctional days of KitKat binges and desktop snoozes.

'Tom, that's all in the past,' said Jo with a smile. 'You weren't well. You weren't in control. But you've turned things around now, and that's all that counts.'

My trusted colleagues had witnessed my lows, so it was only fair that they shared in the highs. In December 2017, when I'd lost my first 50 pounds (23 kilos) in weight – and in doing so reached a physical and emotional milestone – Jo and Sarah were the first people I told. We were walking along a Commons corridor at the time, and I recall looking to my left at Jo, and then looking to my right at Sarah, and noticing their eyes glistening with tears.

'Don't set me off as well,' I said. 'I've got a committee meeting in five minutes' time, and I can't exactly walk in there blubbing, can I?'

As my weight dwindled and my suits sagged, I began to look a bit like Talking Heads' David Byrne in his 'Once in a Lifetime' video. Indeed, following my frontbench appearance at Prime Minister's Questions, a good friend of mine – a Labour Party councillor, Bill Gavan – turned up at my constituency office in West Bromwich bearing two black bin bags.

'Can you make sure Tom Watson gets these?' he asked my bemused staff. 'He looked like he was wearing a six-berth Scout tent at PMQs, and he clearly hasn't got the time to go clothes shopping, so I've dug out some of my old gear for him to wear.'

I really appreciated Bill plundering his wardrobe – his classic suits were a near-perfect fit – and for the next four or five months I turned up to PMQs wearing these stylish, second-hand clothes. When they eventually became too baggy I boxed them up and donated them to a fellow Labour Party member, who had just been diagnosed with type 2 diabetes and who was beginning his own weight-loss journey. The handover gave us the opportunity to sit down over a coffee and talk things through. One good turn deserved another, I reckoned.

Walking around in Bill's snazzy suits had given me a tremendous buzz, but buying my very first off-the-peg suit from Marks & Spencer proved to be a hugely pivotal moment. I had spotted this summery, light-blue linen suit dangling on the sale rail for a bargain £90, and when I'd tried it on I'd felt like a million dollars (my brother Dan had told me how amazing he'd felt when he'd squeezed into a pair of

Levi's 501s for the first time; this was my equivalent). Like a kid desperate to wear his brand new shoes straight away, as soon as I'd paid for the suit I returned to the dressing room and changed back into it, stuffing my other clothes into the M&S carrier bag.

I gave my new blue suit its first public airing at the 2018 Ivor Novello Awards, which took place at the Grosvenor House Hotel. I had been asked to present Billy Bragg with his Outstanding Contribution to British Music award – a great privilege for me, since he was a music hero of mine – and I walked onto the stage feeling on top of the world.

'Billy's political lyrics challenge us,' I said to the assembled audience, 'but his songs of love reach deep into our souls. And for my generation, who have grown up with him from the early beginnings of his career, it is a genuine pleasure to see him recognised by such distinguished colleagues from all sectors of the music industry today.'

The cameras began to click, and Billy and I flashed our smiles. I remember thinking that, for the first time in my life, I didn't have to worry about looking like a sack of spuds in the following day's newspapers.

The print and broadcast media soon began to use my weight loss as an angle for their reports and features, perhaps prompted by a photo that I'd posted for a laugh on my official blog after an engagement in central London.

'One of these is a Neanderthal skeleton held under close security by the Natural History Museum,' I wrote, alongside a picture of me next to this ancient relic. 'The other has lost 86lb in weight.'

Some lobby journalists, many of whom worked under a great deal of pressure and may well have had their own health and lifestyle issues, began to quiz me about the whys and wherefores of my weight-loss journey. What most piqued their curiosity, however, was my Bulletproof Coffee intake. I remember taking part in an interview with the BBC's Nick Robinson for his Political Thinking podcast, and as he kicked off proceedings he proudly presented me with a paper cup of insipid black coffee, complete with a yellow pat of butter floating on the surface. It looked nothing like a bona fide Bulletproof, and it tasted absolutely revolting.

'One lump of butter or two?' he said, laughing, before enquiring how this crazy coffee had curbed my sugar cravings and rid me of my brain fog.

'It's like mainlining saturated fat into your physiology,' I said. 'I just stopped being hungry, Nick, and it's really helped me.'

Tellingly, I chose not to mention my type 2 diabetes diagnosis. Perhaps it was superstition on my part, or maybe even a lingering sense of shame, but until I was certain that I was in long-term remission, and that it wasn't a blip, I thought it wise to keep schtum.

A few weeks later, early one morning, I found myself at Four Millbank, the Westminster-based office block in which many TV companies housed small studios. I visited the cosy little café there, the Atrium, and was delighted to see that they'd started serving proper, blended Bulletproof Coffee, complete with Dave Asprey's Brain Octane Oil.

'Hey, it's fantastic that you're doing this,' I said to the waitress as I ordered my own frothy mugful. 'You must be one of the few places in London that sells it.'

'Well, we've had so many journos requesting this Bulletproof stuff, we thought we'd add it to the menu,' she replied. 'Apparently there's been some MP bloke banging on about it, and everyone wants to know what all the fuss is about.'

I handed over the cash, took receipt of my coffee and allowed myself a little smile.

During the first half of 2018 I remained pretty disciplined with my ketogenic eating programme, but as summer approached I began to relax the parameters and become a little less stringent. I allowed myself to slightly exceed the strict 20g of carbohydrates per day, and followed something more akin to a Mediterranean diet, albeit a loose-ish version without the pasta or the bread (I was pleased to find a great online recipe for a wheat-free loaf made with almond flour). I had no qualms about serving up some brown rice or sweet potato alongside a salmon steak or a chicken breast, although, when my kids weren't looking, I'd often nick a few chips from their plates. Whenever I dined out I'd opt, for example, for a tuna salad with tomatoes and green beans (the tomatoes and the beans were slightly higher on the glycaemic index and weren't strictly keto). These tweaks definitely took me beyond the 20g limit, but I was nowhere near the 150–200g that I'd consumed in the past.

During the summer recess I went on holiday to Italy with Siobhan, the kids and my in-laws, Paul and Karen. The week before we jetted off I had to buy a whole new set of shorts and trunks from my favourite sports outlet in West Bromwich, since the 2017 versions would have fallen down around my ankles, like some fella on a Donald McGill seaside postcard. Compared with bygone holidays, though, this one was a revelation. My new and improved fitness meant that I was able to spend hours in the swimming pool, diving in and splashing around with Malachy and Saoirse – *arrivederci*, flying whale – and, unlike previous years, I was able to comfortably walk around in the heat instead of docking myself permanently on a sunbed.

However, while the kids loved being around their hale and hearty dad, I'm not sure that was the case with the adults. Even though I was on holiday, I was still incredibly mindful of what I ate and drank (far too mindful, in retrospect), since I was very anxious about veering off course and unravelling my good work. When everyone else tucked into some speciality pasta or gelato in a hillside restaurant, for instance, I'd stick to a simple cheese salad or a piece of fruit, before meticulously keying my choices into the MyFitnessPal app. When Paul cracked open some local Italian fizz back at the villa, I'd politely decline and continue sipping my iced water, before retiring to bed with my latest nutritional science book for company.

I had developed a deep-seated fear of letting myself go and, because of this, most evenings I must have been duller than ditchwater. Siobhan and her parents had the good grace to avoid making this an issue, though, but as the week went by I think they probably missed the old Tom, that party-loving bon viveur who liked a drink, a song and a slice (or six) of pizza.

Back home in the UK, my obsessive behaviour began to irritate my good pal David, too. While he'd been extremely supportive in the past ('It's amazing what you've done, Tom, you're just like a normal fat bloke, now,' he'd said in his broad West Yorkshire accent when I'd lost that first 50lb or 23 kilos), I think my born-again health and fitness fixation soon became a little wearing. During our walks around Kennington Park he'd raise his eyes skywards as I eulogised about a book I'd read, or a podcast I'd found, and would often pointedly ignore me or tetchily change the subject.

'Honestly, David, you've got to check out this link,' I'd say. 'It'll blow your mind.'

'I don't need to check it out, Tom,' he'd wearily reply. 'You've told me twice already.'

David may disagree, but I think the dynamics between us began to change when I overtook him, weight-wise. I had always been the Ollie to his Stan, the Large to his Little, and when I finally became lighter than him, effectively passing him on the way down, I sensed some friction between us. Our trips to the pub soon became fewer and further between (especially when I started to resist the temptation of downing pints as a reward for a fitness goal) and, as we sensed ourselves drifting apart, we soon stopped walking together.

Much of the blame probably lay with me. Having restored my health and reclaimed my mojo, I'd probably become a little self-absorbed and had no doubt bored my mate into submission. But this particular predicament also demonstrated how relationships could change and evolve following a major life event, be that marriage, divorce, illness, childbirth or, yes, even weight loss. It was inevitable, I suppose, that my friendship dynamics would shift, and that my social diary would shrink. Going out for beer, curry and a late-night karaoke session with my mates Kevin Brennan, Ian Lucas and Michael Dugher – known in parliamentary circles as 'the choir' – soon became a thing of the past, and I also found myself declining invitations to various parties and gatherings.

Perhaps a pared-down social life was unavoidable in my circumstances. Looking back, if there was any downside to my personal health journey, this was probably it.

During the summer of 2018 I began to consider the prospect of going public about my type 2 diabetes. My thinking was largely prompted by a meeting I had with a man called Dan Parker who worked in partnership with Jamie Oliver's organisation, helping to promote its healthy eating campaign for children. He happened to mention that he was a type 2 diabetic – I chose not to divulge my own diagnosis – and we struck up a conversation about the perils of the sugar economy. The sugar tax had been implemented earlier that year (the only good thing George Osborne ever did as chancellor of the exchequer) and I was becoming increasingly interested in challenging 'Big Sugar' interests. Dan proceeded to tell me his own T2D story, explaining how his illness caused him much embarrassment – he often felt like a failure – and how he reckoned he wasn't alone in that respect.

'In a room full of a hundred people, maybe ten to fifteen per cent of them will have type 2 diabetes,' he said. 'Ask those people to raise their hand, and only one or two people will, because the others feel so damned ashamed.'

As far as Dan was concerned, this stigma prevailed throughout society. T2D was a badge of guilt, almost, and in order to rectify this, and to help people address and improve their condition, much more openness and awareness was required.

His remarks played on my mind for weeks – I too had suffered those same feelings of shame and isolation – and I soon concluded that it was time for me to speak openly and publicly about my health journey. I worked with my Westminster team to locate a suitable occasion and, with this in mind, we set up a meeting with ukactive, a not-for-profit organisation that existed to improve the health of the nation through fitness and movement. They were intrigued to hear my story and very kindly invited me to speak at their national summit, scheduled for 12 September 2018. My colleagues and I then began the creative process of writing a speech. Usually a speech involves a three-way collaboration between myself and my press team, who ensure the right number of media hooks, and my policy team, who try to make it strategy-rich. However, since this particular speech was intensely personal, I wrote most of it myself, and wrote it from the heart.

My press officer, Sarah Coombes, formulated a comprehensive PR strategy to accompany my announcement. Throughout the morning I would attend a number of radio, television and newspaper interviews, including a primetime slot on ITV's *Good Morning Britain*. I knew for a fact that many Westminster politicians disliked appearing on *GMB*, fearing the programme's notoriously tough interviews. The combative Piers Morgan and the forensic Susanna Reid were indeed a formidable duo – I'd seen many a guest shrink as they received a breakfast-time grilling – but I'd always enjoyed the experience. I liked sparring with Piers, and I admired Susanna's incisive line of questioning.

I awoke at 4.30 that morning, and within the hour a *GMB* car had dropped me off at their White City studios. I walked into the make-up room, and received a warm welcome from Piers, Susanna and the production team.

'Bloody hell, Tom, you're half the man you used to be,' said Piers, grinning. 'Fair play to you, sir.'

'Cheers, Piers,' I replied.

I went on air at 7.30 a.m., and Susanna opened the interview by expressing her astonishment at my weight loss.

'It's remarkable,' she said. 'Your physical presence has changed. Seven stone is a massive amount to lose. How have you done it?'

'Well, I really did it by completely changing my diet,' I replied. 'I cut out all refined sugar and high-sugar foods, and then I started exercising. There's no secret code.'

I told Susanna how I considered myself a reformed sugar addict, and how I'd come to realise that my entire diet had been based around grazing on sweet things. Sugar addiction was a real illness, I said, and it was one of the reasons why the country was facing a huge obesity crisis.

'I started like everyone else, a middle-aged guy in his fifties, trying to get the weight off, and at my biggest I was twenty-two stone,' I added. 'I read the work of Dr Michael Mosley, and then I read *The Pioppi Diet*, and they both were, in many senses, contradicting the advice we're given by health experts in government. So I then read the footnotes, and read all the scientific papers, because I needed to understand what was going on with my own body.'

Piers then quizzed me about my exercise regime, and I responded by saying that, despite physical activity being an instrumental part of my turnaround, the most important factor had been my diet.

'When guys get really overweight and decide to attack it, the first thing they do is join a gym, and they never sort their nutrition out,' I said. 'I would say to people, if you don't sort your nutrition out, there's virtually no point in doing exercise.'

'Abs are made in the kitchen,' said Susanna with a wink.

'I can't quite see my abs yet.' I laughed.

A producer then entered the studio carrying a tray of Bulletproof Coffees (the genuine article, nothing like the BBC aberration), which prompted Piers to switch into rant mode.

'Here's this infamous thing that you've revealed that you take, and that you swear by. I've got to say it looks *disgusting,*' he sneered, before taking a sip. 'OK, it tastes like a creamy lattè, but what is the point of Bulletproof Coffee?'

I told him that, in the early days, slightly upping my fat intake had helped me to quell my sugar cravings and that a cup of the stuff could often see me through until lunchtime. That seemed to answer his question, because the conversation swiftly turned to my day job. Piers demanded my views on the Labour Party's Brexit proposals, accusing my fellow colleagues of a lack of clarity and condemning us for apparently sitting on the fence. Things got a bit testy and ill-tempered as I attempted to argue our cause.

'Perhaps you're the wrong guy to use this phrase with, Tom, but that's like having your cake and eating it,' yelled Piers. 'You probably haven't had cake in a year.'

'You can get as angry as you want about it,' I retorted. 'Maybe *you* should try taking less sugar in your Bulletproof Coffee.'

Like I said, I enjoyed the occasional duel with Piers.

There was one question, though, that Susanna had been dying to ask me, but had dared not address while we were on air. She hadn't been the first person to pose it; it was a topic that had aroused the interest of others, too.

'Not wishing to sound rude, Tom, but do you have saggy skin?' she'd whispered during an advert break. 'It can be one of the downsides of rapid weight loss, can't it?'

'It can,' I replied, unperturbed, 'but I've been pretty lucky in that respect.'

I told her that, while I didn't possess a defined chest or a washboard stomach (there'd always be a certain amount of middle-age padding), at the same time I didn't have rolls of skin hanging off me. Perhaps my skin elasticity was in the genes, I suggested, although there may well have been other factors. I had read somewhere that rubbing a magnesium-based cream supplement into your skin could be advantageous, so I'd given that a try, and I'd also listened with interest to a Dr Jason Fung podcast that highlighted the potential benefits of intermittent fasting in this regard. Fasting apparently helped to promote a condition called autophagy (which involved the body flushing out damaged cells before renewing healthy cells) and many of Dr Fung's patients who'd pursued that route had tended to avoid excess skin issues.

'I occasionally tried that as well,' I explained to Susanna, 'although I can't be totally sure that it made any difference.'

'Thank you for answering my very cheeky question,' she said, smiling, as the ad break finished and the cameras began to roll again.

Later that afternoon, at Westminster's Queen Elizabeth II conference centre, I stood at the lectern, ready to deliver my keynote speech at the ukactive summit. Sitting behind me on the stage were Dame Tanni Grey-Thompson, the former Paralympian and chair of the organisation, and Andrew Lansley, the former health secretary who'd once governed – or should that be tried to govern – the NHS. Facing me in the auditorium were hundreds of the UK's finest fitness professionals, most of whom would have known what a health journey looked like, and would have worked with plenty of fat, fifty-something blokes like me in their gyms.

In my line of work I'd attended hundreds of speaking engagements, but this time around I felt unusually nervous, and quite vulnerable. That morning I'd opened up about my weight-loss journey on *Good Morning Britain* but here, on this public platform, before an audience of strangers, I was about to reveal for the first time the full extent of my illness.

'Since last summer, I've lost ninety-nine pounds in weight. The pounds have flown off me almost as quickly as they've flown off local government public health budgets,' I said, as I imagined Andrew Lansley giving me the side-eye.

'There was a personal reason why I realised I had to take action with my own health, though,' I continued. 'I was diagnosed a few years back with type 2 diabetes. I'm not unusual. There are 3.8 million adults in the UK with diabetes, 90 per cent of them with type 2, which is more than twice as many as there were twenty years ago.

'But I'm pleased and very relieved to say that, thanks to a quite radical change of diet and behaviour – not just exercising more, but eradicating ultra-processed food, fast food, starchy carbs and refined sugar – my own type 2 diabetes is in remission. I am no longer taking medication for it, and I feel absolutely *fantastic*.

'But what I know now, that I didn't know when I was first diagnosed, is that type 2 diabetes can be prevented. I'm living proof that it can be put into remission, and that's my central message today. We have to get better as a country at doing both: prevention and remission. Yet too many people today have no clue that their condition can be beaten, and I'd like to send a simple message to all the other type 2 diabetes sufferers, all three million of them. I believe in remission for all. The vast majority of those people with type 2 diabetes can get off their medication with the right combination of nutrition and exercise, and that's the task for all of us in this room. If they do, they will live longer and more fulfilling lives.'

I then suggested a few tweaks to the government's public health policy – irking Andrew Lansley, no doubt – before bringing my speech to a close by praising the good work of ukactive, and by pledging my ongoing support.

The reception I received was heartening – the applause from these top-notch professionals meant a great deal – and afterwards I was approached by a string of delegates offering me their thanks and good wishes.

'Thank you, Tom,' said a leisure manager from Greater Manchester who came over to shake my hand. 'We see lots of success stories in our jobs, but it's always great when someone in the public eye can share their own positive experience. Raising awareness like this can have such a huge impact, and can really help to inspire others.'

'Well, you never know, maybe one day I could train up to become a gym instructor in my spare time,' I said, grinning.

He perked up at this, telling me that the industry recognised that there was a dearth of instructors of a 'certain age' who could offer well-placed advice and genuine empathy to fellow forty- and fifty-something gym-goers. With this in mind, organisations needed to provide a more inclusive and understanding environment, and as such needed to recruit staff from all age ranges.

Mmm, I thought. *I quite like the idea of that.*

When I returned to my Westminster office I was greeted by my press officer, Sarah, who'd been tasked with monitoring my social media throughout the day. She had also posted up a short video on Twitter and Facebook that outlined my new mission to help others and reiterated the Labour Party's commitment to halting the alarming rise of type 2 diabetes.

'Tom, it's gone absolutely crazy,' she said. 'Over two thousand retweets on Twitter, ten thousand likes, and hundreds of responses on the Facebook page. Come and have a look.'

I leaned over her computer and scrolled through the tweets:

> @tom_watson Great campaign. Importantly, it acknowledges that it's not just the fault of the individual. We're all being lied to by the food industry, there should be much tighter regulation on how much sugar is put in foods, how it's marketed.

> @tom_watson Low carbohydrate is what countless cardiologists and doctors have been advocating for many, many years and yet the naysayers are doing their best to 'prove' them wrong. Long live the movement for cutting down on starchy and sugary carbs. Well done Tom

@tom_watson Well done on your progress against diabetes Tom, and I wish you all the very best for the future, including, I hope, in government promoting this health message in a way that has been sadly absent under the current administration.

@tom_watson You are an inspirational role model & superb example of how we can change our habits, our lives and our health for the better. Thank you & very well done.

@tom_watson With you all the way on this. There needs to be government intervention on the disproportionately high cost and limited availability of fresh foods, funded by a tax on sugar and multinationals that profit from junk food.

@tom_watson Well done, that's fantastic. As a food teacher I spend a lot of time teaching about healthy eating and teaching healthy recipes, hopefully together we can help with improving the health of the nation.

@tom_watson When you increase your intake of healthy fats and lower your carbs (from my experience) the cravings subside. It does take discipline and a proactive approach to your health and longevity. I'm proof, along with Tom, that it works.

Some of them raised a smile, too:

@tom_watson Quite astonishing how much you now resemble Eddie Mair.

@tom_watson Oh great. Now I'll never be able to tell him and Elvis Costello apart.

@tom_watson You can legitimately wear Fred Perry polos again.

Over on Facebook, the positive (and not-so-positive) comments rained in, too:

I lost 4.5st cutting out processed sugars and doing moderate exercise. Good luck with your mission, people don't realise it's an addictive substance until they try and come off it...

Saw you on GMB this morning. Inspirational! Great to hear your views about sugar addiction too. Have a feeling I'd find it hard to wean myself off it! People don't realise how addictive it is.

Big congrats Tom, I've been on a similar journey. Odd how things stick in the mind, my happiest time was being able to buy a suit from M&S rather the local big man's shop!

I did it that way too. Lost 7 stones and I am off medication and in a normal blood range. All within 18 months. It's great to see someone speak up about it. Well done.

A great role model for men of a certain age and shape. Well done!

Tom, you have lost more than my wife weighs! Congratulations and I applaud your campaign.

Dear Tom – I'm a Conservative through and through, but am just coming here in the spirit of doing something different on Facebook than attack the other side. I really salute your efforts and dedication to your health and well-being – it's really inspirational and I hope a great example of what can be achieved. All the best to you.

Amazing Poster Boy – well done Tom, and good luck with helping everyone to improve their health in the UK.

Tom: a real achievement and genuinely worthy of admiration. All you have to do now is give up the capitalist status quo and embrace genuine democratic socialism.

Brilliant work, Tom! No one can accuse the socialists of not having the ambition to better themselves. Now it's official, a very positive message.

Brilliant. Lose the sugar, the poison of the body. Then lose neoliberalism, the poison of the socialist mind.

I admire what you are doing but I once only ever voted Labour but since commies took over never again and you stick up for them.

On the whole (and with the exception of a few trolls and naysayers) I was showered with goodwill in the months following my revelation, and was often waylaid on the street by people wishing me well or asking for advice. I was always careful when I did this, though, prefacing everything I said with some precautionary words.

'Look, I can only say how I've done it,' I remember telling a hefty bloke in his forties who'd approached me in West Bromwich's Queen's Square Shopping Centre. 'That might not necessarily be the way you should do it, though. There's no one-size-fits-all. Sometimes you need to plot your own journey.'

I received hundreds of emails from members of the public – I tried my best to reply to them all, often pointing them in the direction of different books, websites and pieces of research – and I was also sent some kind messages from one or two celebrities, including a very famous TV presenter. Also making contact via Twitter was the actor Nick Frost, who was best known for starring with Simon Pegg in *Hot Fuzz* and *Shaun of the Dead*, and who was often accused of being my doppelgänger.

'I wish you'd have run this past me first,' he tweeted, having seen a post about my slimmed-down self. 'This has severely dented my chances of playing you in any future biopic. My only hope is the film takes place before the dramatic weight loss.'

Nick's wasn't the only amusing response to my transformation. Toward the end of 2018 my cartoonist nemesis, the *Guardian*'s Steve Bell, created a new moniker for me. I was now Fatberg Slim, still glowering behind my black-rimmed glasses, but now sporting a leaner frame and a smaller suit. My feelings about it were mixed, I suppose. While part of me grudgingly respected the way he'd segued from his original caricature – give him his dues, it was very clever – the other part of me gained some private pleasure that my previous incarnation was no longer relevant. The Fatberg, version 1.0, was history.

CHAPTER SIX

Channelling My Mind, Challenging My Body

In November 2018 I had the honour of being interviewed by Dave Asprey. He had got wind that a British MP had been extolling the virtues of his Bulletproof Coffee over in the UK, and had very kindly invited me onto his podcast to share my own weight-loss story with his army of subscribers. It was a genuine privilege.

'He's sitting here on Skype looking like a picture of health, not like a guy who was seven stone heavier than he is now,' said Dave in his introduction. 'We're going to talk about how he did it and what it's going to take to get the government to help all of us be a little nicer to each other.'

'I'm incredibly grateful to be speaking with you,' I replied, 'because you've had such an impact on my life. You've actually sent me in a whole new direction. It's great to be talking to your listeners, too, because I know that they've either been through the experience that we've been through, or they're about to, and their lives are transformed. It's a great feeling.'

Dave and I covered a wide range of topics, putting the world to rights about the scale of the diabetes time-bomb in the UK and the power of the 'big food' corporations in the

US. On a more personal note, we discussed our individual approaches to mental and physical well-being, whereupon I explained that I'd entered into stage two of my lifestyle plan. Ditching the sugar and changing my diet had helped me to shed the weight, clear my head and bin my metformin, but mine was definitely an ongoing project. There remained many physical and emotional refinements on my to-do list.

'I've only just started,' I told Dave.

Despite being a churchgoer (my lifestyle changes and realigned priorities had brought me even closer to my Christian faith), I probably read more about other religions than my own. I became particularly fascinated with Buddhism, more out of academic interest than anything, and often referred to a pair of fabulous books on the subject, *Buddhism for Beginners* by Jack Kornfield and *The Joy of Living* by Yongey Mingyur Rinpoche.

I found myself being increasingly drawn to the Buddhist principle of 'right-mindfulness'. This therapeutic technique is an integral component of the 'eight-fold path' toward happiness and fulfilment, and is all about attuning yourself to your emotions, and appreciating your environment. It is a concept that allows you to focus on the here and now by reconnecting with your body's feelings, listening to your inner dialogue and detaching yourself from the material things in life. By becoming alive to the moment, and by gaining control of your thoughts, you're less likely to worry about the past or the future and are more able to value the present.

Practising complete mindfulness – centring myself, if you will – is quite a skill, and it took some getting used to. One technique involved listening to all the ambient noise around me, focusing first on the farthest sound (maybe an aeroplane, or some distant traffic) and then gradually zoning in on something much closer, maybe some birdsong, or even my own breathing rhythm. Occasionally I'd start my day with five minutes of silent meditation, reclining on a chair in the corner of my lounge, concentrating on all the sensations in my body, from my head down to my toes. I discovered that this short period of calm reflection set me up for the rest of the day, enabling me to curb that primitive, adrenaline-fuelled fight-or-flight response that had often afflicted me at Westminster. For more structured mindfulness, I also began to use the Headspace app. Its bite-sized, guided meditation sessions became truly life-enhancing for me, covering themes from sleep and anxiety to stress and motivation.

Conforming to a more contemplative mindset aided other areas of my life, too. Along with the wise counsel of Aristotle – his 'we are what we repeatedly do' maxim was still firmly affixed to my fridge door – I became a creature of routine, organising my life in such a way that I had fewer obstructions and distractions to derail me. Two books I read were instrumental in this respect: *Aristotle's Way* by renowned classicist Edith Hall, which brought the ancient philosopher to life, coupled with

Atomic Habits, a *New York Times* bestseller written by entrepreneur James Clear.

Part of Clear's study focused on cycling supremo Dave Brailsford, outlining his belief that success lies in the aggregation of marginal gains. Brailsford believes that the cumulative application of tweaks and refinements, no matter how minuscule, can – over time – have positive, long-term consequences. He therefore had cycle tyres painted with alcohol, for instance, so they'd gain a little more traction on the road. Riders wore heated over-shorts, so their muscles would feel slightly warmer. Mattresses and pillows were carefully tested, in order to optimise competitors' sleep.

Clear's own theory about habits and change also fascinated me. As he saw it, there existed three levels of behavioural change.

He wrote:

> The first layer is changing your outcomes. This level is concerned with changing your results: losing weight, publishing a book, winning a championship. Most of the goals you set are associated with this level of change.
>
> The second layer is changing your process. This level is concerned with changing your habits and systems: implementing a new routine at the gym, decluttering your desk for better workflow, developing a meditation practice. Most of the habits you build are associated with this level.

The third and deepest layer is changing your identity. This level is concerned with changing your beliefs: your worldview, your self-image, your judgements about yourself and others. Most of the beliefs, assumptions, and biases you hold are associated with this level.

Many people, said Clear, start the process of change by focusing on what they want to achieve, which leads to outcome-based habits. The alternative is to focus on who we wish to become, by building identity-based habits.

His words really struck a chord. In many ways, I still saw myself as a fat bloke who was just trying to lose weight. Instead, I needed to start habitually thinking of myself as a fit bloke who, through diet and exercise, was striving to attain health and happiness.

As a result of my further reading, my day-to-day routines became far more streamlined and automatic. Channelling the Dave Brailsford approach of control and micromanagement, I implemented various life rules that simplified the low-level decisions that I made on a daily basis. Something as fundamental as designating a special place for my trainers helped to declutter my mind and instil some order. For thirty years I'd flung them into a random dark corner, after which I'd wasted valuable time trying to find the darned things, and then wasted more mental energy by berating myself for my slovenliness.

I bought myself a set of colour-coded notepads, too, so I could embed 'to-do' lists into my ritual. These action points, related to both home and work matters, enabled me to better sequence my life, thus muting the cacophony of internal voices that had often nagged me to do this, that and everything.

I also decided to keep a 'gratitude journal', having been given the idea by a friend. At the end of each day, I aimed to write down two or three sentences that made me feel thankful and optimistic, whether it was a small act of kindness shown to me by a colleague, or a beautiful sunset that I'd seen over Westminster. I also used this journal to encourage my own positive deeds and actions, perhaps prompting myself to drop a thank-you note to an intern for assisting me with some research, or reminding myself to ring a Labour Party councillor who'd been suffering with ill-health.

I tried to implant mindfulness elements into my day-to-day work life, too. The Brexit crisis had caused a great amount of stress among MPs across the board, with one Tory MP even claiming that he'd escaped the political turmoil by hiding in a dark Commons cupboard. I did my utmost to keep myself on an even keel, though, stealing a few moments of calm, solitary reflection whenever the pressure began to mount (the Headspace app often helped in this regard) and avoiding any altercations with colleagues regarding this hugely divisive subject. Naturally, I had very strong views on Brexit – I'd always publicly supported a second referendum – but I also respected fellow members whose opinions were diametrically opposed to mine. My friend and fellow Labour MP, Gloria De Piero, was extremely committed to delivering Brexit in light of the June 2016 result. A number of pro-Remain colleagues reacted with disgust, and virtually excommunicated her, but I refused to let any political differences affect our relationship.

'We've been friends for thirty years, Gloria,' I said when we spoke over the phone one evening. 'Why on earth would I want to fall out with you over this?'

'Seems you're in the minority, though, Tom,' she replied.

During the Brexit debates of 2019, I'd look around the Commons and witness MPs almost foaming at the mouth, their faces puce with rage as they hurled insults at opponents (indeed, a few years earlier, in the midst of my sugar addiction, I might well have been that person). I remember sitting in the febrile atmosphere of the chamber, wondering whether calmer mindsets and deeper thoughts might have encouraged more collaborative discourse and less spite and recrimination. Who knows? Had more Westminster folk embraced mindfulness, perhaps our country might have been coaxed out of the Brexit mire in a more timely and dignified fashion.

As the Brexi-shambles rumbled on, achieving quality downtime in London and the Midlands became more important than ever before, though now that I was feeling much healthier and happier, I found myself yearning less for the company of others. In my twenties, thirties and forties, I'd always needed to be where the action was, pressing the flesh at Commons receptions or partying with friends in a Frith Street drinking den. In contrast, the arrival of my fifties saw me craving solitude, and purposely spending more time alone in my little one-bedroom London flat. Turning my life around had encouraged me to like myself a lot more, I guess, and I'd genuinely started to appreciate my own company. Without sounding like a mad old hermit, my reflective outlook and my newfound clear-headedness allowed me to strike up meaningful conversations with myself, and I'd happily sit alone in my living room, mulling over issues and dreaming up ideas.

During my spare time in London I found myself listening to things for entertainment, rather than watching them; other than audiobooks (both fiction and non-fiction) my devices were forever streaming podcasts (notably those appertaining to health, poetry and philosophy) and my digital radio dial flitted between BBC Radio 4, LBC and BBC 6 Music. Spotify and BBC Sounds fulfilled my enduring love of music, too, enabling me to switch effortlessly between rock and pop, and between indie and classical, allowing me to fill my flat with Led Zeppelin one morning, and Kylie Minogue the next. I loved their curated playlists, too, particularly BBC Sounds' Mindfulness Mix. Somebody once told me that the antidote to loneliness was solitude, not sociability, and – even though it took me five decades to realise it – I believe this is spot on. There have been times when I've felt lonelier in parliament, surrounded by people, than I have done in my flat, on my own.

My priorities and my perspective have indeed altered of late, and my work–life balance has shifted. I don't find the all-consuming nature of politics a particularly rewarding endeavour any more. While I respect the institution of parliament, and I admire (most of) my fellow politicians, the daily skirmishes and the constant in-fighting, particularly since the summer of 2016, has been wearing and demoralising. I can't deny that my transformational health journey has changed me as a person, has given me a much deeper sense of what really matters and has provided me with a whole new outlook. Of paramount importance to me, of course, is that my children are happy and healthy, that they are kind and compassionate and that they appreciate the people and the world around them. I deeply regret that, in the early days of my political career, I didn't devote enough time and attention to Malachy and Saoirse; nowadays I go to extraordinary lengths to ensure that I'm present in their lives, zigzagging across the country if necessary.

My close friends and family are more important to me than ever before, too – they're a very loyal and supportive bunch – and I hope that, as time has passed, and as my life has changed, I've become a better ally to them: more helpful, more thoughtful, more mindful.

It is sometimes said that the four pillars of good health are nutrition, exercise, well-being and sleep; from my experience, though, you can build the first three on the latter. My sleep problems began around the same time as I was elected as an MP. Whether it was attending late-night votes in the Commons, enjoying midnight meals in curry houses or staying in stuffy hotel rooms during campaigns, I was lucky to snatch five hours per night, six at most. Looking back, my ill-disciplined sleep had a pretty disastrous impact upon my health, and I remain convinced that my disrupted circadian rhythm contributed to my insulin resistance, my high blood pressure and, ultimately, my obesity.

In those days, my final act before hitting the sack was to check the #TomorrowsPapersToday hashtag on Twitter, just in case there were any front-page stories that needed my immediate attention (if so, I'd invariably fire off an early-hours email to alert my staff). Then, after experiencing a fitful night's sleep – broken by at least two toilet trips – I'd wake up feeling achy and disorientated, groaning in pain and barely able to remember what day it was. Tellingly, the first deed of the morning wasn't to clamber out of bed for a stretch, or grab a glass of water from the kitchen; it was to fumble for my phone in order to check the Labour Party's overnight media briefing. This missive would reach my phone between 4 a.m. and 6 a.m., the expectation being that we MPs would digest it before breakfast.

I soon came to realise that my night-time health needed as much attention as my daytime health. I sought help and guidance from a brilliant book, *Why We Sleep: The New Science of Sleep and Dreams* by Matthew Walker, Professor of Neuroscience and Psychology at the University of California. The conclusions he drew, in both his book and online broadcasts, were absolutely fascinating.

'Sleep is emotional first aid,' he said. 'Sleep is the greatest life support system that you could ever wish for.

Sleep de-risks nearly every disease in the Western world.'

I was particularly intrigued by the chapter titled 'What's Stopping You from Sleeping?' in which Walker identified the perils of electric light around bedtime. He spoke eloquently about this in interviews, too.

'Man-made light began the re-engineering of sleep patterns with the invention of gas lamps,' he explained. 'When darkness arrives, the body is flooded with melatonin that prepares us for sleep. Electric light tricks your suprachiasmatic nucleus, which fools your brain into thinking the sun hasn't set. So we go to bed when our body is not biologically capable of sleep.

'Light receptors in the eye are most sensitive to short-wavelength blue LED light. It has twice the harmful impact on melatonin suppression. An iPad used two hours before bed can block melatonin by nearly a quarter.' He went on to quote a study that found that reading books on an iPad, rather than print books, suppressed melatonin release by up to half and delayed production by as much as three hours, with the result that those taking part lost REM sleep, reported broken sleep and had reduced melatonin production for days afterwards.

Reading Professor Walker's book became my catalyst for change, and from then on I tried to ring-fence at least eight hours per night for sleep. This wasn't always feasible with my work schedule, but wherever possible I aimed to be tucked up in bed between 9 p.m. and 10 p.m., with my alarm set for 6 a.m. at the latest. To provide a sleep-friendly environment, I ensured that my bedroom was clutter-free, that it was suitably dark (thick curtains, tightly closed) and that it had a pleasantly ambient temperature. I banned myself from looking at any form of electronic device for an hour before bedtime (and for an hour after waking) and even bought myself a pair of blue-light-blocking glasses to reduce any screen glare at other times of the day. While I kept a phone on my bedside table at night, just in case any emergency calls came in from my kids, or from work, I never accessed social media or surfed the net. I also stopped scrolling through the daily media brief at silly o'clock, finally realising that it was a wholly inadequate way to start the day. Instead, I addressed any important issues once I arrived at the office. If there was something that I needed to respond to urgently, I could count on my team to inform me as soon as I walked through the door.

In order to monitor my sleep patterns (and to satisfy my geeky obsession with stats and gadgets) I invested in a brilliant little device called an Oura Ring. Worn on your middle finger, it digitally tracks your sleep activity (as well as your pulse, your body temperature and your heart rate) and it was a total revelation. I learned, for example, that if I drank just one glass of wine with my evening meal, my resting heart rate would increase by about ten beats per minute. Also, if I ate later than 6 p.m., my sleep would be much more disturbed and erratic than normal, particularly during the REM (rapid eye movement) phase, which stimulates the brain regions used in learning, memory and mood. If the Oura Ring showed an unusual rise in overnight body temperature, I surmised that I'd trained too hard in the gym that day, and would be inclined to tone things down the next. This powerful diagnostic tool soon became an indispensable part of my well-being plan, and I found myself extolling its virtues to countless friends and colleagues.

'This thing's amazing. Couldn't do without it,' I said to my friend Peter Mandelson, who'd shown a keen interest in my new gadget when we'd caught up for a coffee one afternoon.

'How fascinating…' drawled the man I often playfully refer to as The Dark Lord.

With my enhanced night-time schedule, I finally learned to love mornings. No longer did I wake up with a jolt, my bones creaky, my skin clammy. Instead I opened my eyes and allowed myself to come slowly to my senses, feeling renewed and refreshed following an unbroken eight-hour kip. I would then put on my trainers and go for my customary walk in Kennington Park, or perhaps along the South Bank, in order to stretch my legs and to absorb some early-morning daylight. Having read a compelling book penned by another sleep expert – Satchin Panda's *The Circadian Code* – I had learned that taking a thirty-minute walk after sunrise could have a huge impact on the synchronisation of your body clock. Allowing light onto your skin and into the backs of your eyes at that time of day could effectively help your brain to understand that, when the sun set and the skies darkened, it was time for your body to prepare for sleep.

As someone whose sleep patterns have been transformed, I cannot emphasise enough the importance of a good night's shut-eye. Sadly, research shows that too many people in the UK are suffering with sleep deprivation, which can have severe implications for their health and well-being, whether it's increasing the risk of strokes, heart disease and hypertension or prompting conditions like anxiety and depression.

A Royal Society for Public Health survey in 2016 found that the average sleep time was 6.8 hours, below the 7.7 hours that people thought they needed (the RSPH also called for the UK government to publish a national sleep strategy). The following year, the Sleep Council carried out a survey of 5,000 people in Great Britain and found that 74 per cent of Brits slept less than seven hours per night, that 30 per cent experienced poor sleep most nights and that the top three reasons for poor sleep were stress and worry, partner disturbance and noise.

Organisations like the Sleep Council are doing sterling work to promote sleep awareness, but I still think there's plenty more to be done by key policymakers. I believe we all have the right to eight hours' uninterrupted rest per night, and I'd fully endorse a public health campaign designed to restore people's sleep patterns and to enhance their well-being. Perhaps we could liaise more closely with urban house builders and property developers, requesting that they include soundproofed windows and blackout blinds in every bedroom as standard. Maybe we could look at amending employment law, so as to provide added protection for night staff and shift workers. We could also have conversations with senior educators regarding the possibility of implementing later school start times, in recognition of the fact that adolescents have different circadian rhythms (yes, there's an evolutionary reason why they lie in). Every one of us deserves the freedom to sleep; it's central to our well-being, and forms the bedrock for good health.

In the latter part of 2018, as alluded to in my podcast chat with Dave Asprey, I began to ramp up my physical fitness. I had been continuing my boxercise and cardiovascular training with Clayton (either in Kennington Park or his Bermondsey gym, depending on the weather), but there came a point when I decided to mix things up a bit, and introduce some weight training into my regular routine. I had whittled myself down to 15 stone (95 kilos), which I was inordinately happy about, but I felt like I was plateauing, and that there was still more work to be done and more weight to be lost. I had read up on the benefits of slow-movement resistance training for middle-aged blokes like me, who, with the right advice and guidance, could increase their basic strength and look and feel better. Beyond that, I also learned that weight-bearing exercise could improve bone and muscle density, thus reducing the risk of osteoporosis (fragile bones) and sarcopenia (muscle loss) among older adults. While these conditions were fairly uncommon among men of my age, putting in the groundwork as a fifty-something could well pay dividends in the future.

I amassed a mini-library of books on the subject. My favourite bedside read, believe it or not, was Arnold

Schwarzenegger's *New Encyclopedia of Modern Bodybuilding* (so weighty was this tome, I needed Arnie-style brawn to lift it). A step-by-step manual of strength training, written in a clear, no-nonsense style, it was the perfect starter-guide for a curious beginner like me. Other books that I found particularly useful included *Body by Science* by Dr Doug McGuff and *Designing Resistance Training Programs* by Steven Fleck and William Kraemer, although these titles were marginally more scholarly.

Furnished with information – and convinced that this was the right course of action – I began to cast around for a suitable gym. In order to fit in with my chock-a-block diary it needed to be as near to my flat as possible, and available to use 24/7, so I plumped for a £34-a-month membership with Snap Fitness in Elephant & Castle. It fitted the bill perfectly. Not only was I able to access an impressive array of lifting equipment (as well as a variety of running machines if rain ever stopped play outdoors), I was also buddied up with an extremely knowledgeable instructor, Nic Cornelis. I attended a few sessions with him in which he showed me the ropes and taught me the basics, explaining how to use each piece of equipment as safely and as efficiently as possible.

'Have to say, I'm a bit nervous about this,' I said, as I eyed a huge set of dumb-bells.

'Don't worry about anything,' replied Nic. 'I won't push you to do anything you can't do.'

It was a daunting experience – I was well outside my comfort zone, and strength and conditioning was never going to come naturally to me – but within a couple of weeks I was pumping iron and lifting weights (and engaging in a few vanity biceps and triceps curls, as you do), although my squats and bench-presses were decidedly amateurish.

By spring 2019 I felt significantly fitter and stronger. Indeed, I'd become so obsessional and evangelical about my new discipline that I'd begun to seriously contemplate getting myself qualified as a part-time Level Two gym instructor, through which I could gain more knowledge about physiology and gym equipment. With this in mind I decided to upgrade to a specialist health club, Ultimate Performance in Mayfair, signing up for one of their two-month programmes with a view to getting myself as toned up (and as genned up) as possible, as well as learning from some of the best trainers in the business. I chose this particular gym for two reasons; firstly, on the strength of its charismatic owner, Nick Mitchell, a highly respected figure in the fitness industry whose book, *The Principles of Muscle Building Program Design*, I'd devoured in one weekend. Ultimate Performance had also been recommended to me by a female colleague at Westminster who, after joining up, had shed a significant amount of weight. Having completely reconditioned her body, she'd successfully completed the London Marathon.

'It's a gym I really can't afford, to get a body I really don't deserve,' I told her once I'd signed on the dotted line in mid-May.

'It'll be well worth it, Tom, I can assure you,' she'd replied. 'The staff there are amazing.'

I was assigned to a personal trainer called Jay, who quizzed me about my long-term goals.

'To carry two bags of shopping up a flight of stairs when I'm an OAP, and to pick up my great-great-grandchildren without slipping a disc,' I said. 'Oh, and to live until I'm 102.'

'Interesting,' he said with a smile, 'although I was kind of thinking about where you wanted to be in three months' time.'

I wanted resistance training to strengthen my body and accelerate my weight loss, I told Jay, and I wanted to be able to walk into any gym in the UK and use any piece of equipment competently and confidently. I also made known my ambition to teach skills to others of a certain age.

'First and foremost, it's all about technique and form, Tom,' said Jay. Technique, he explained, was the manner in which you lifted weights; the positions you adopted, for example, and the movements that you incorporated. Form was the consistency of maintaining those techniques, regardless of speed or weight-load. According to Jay, heeding these fundamentals was far more important than counting repetitions and lifting the heaviest weights possible. All too often, however, both were overlooked by poorly informed gym-goers. They ended up virtually flinging the weights around, which not only trained the wrong muscles, but also increased the risk of potential injury.

'When you're lifting a squat bar, I'll be looking closely at your whole muscle range, so that I can spot and remedy any weaknesses,' said Jay. 'What you do with your abdominals is just as important as what you do with your shoulders.'

Under Jay's expert tutelage, I focused on that all-important form and technique and learned how best to condition my body. Within weeks I began to see the fruits of my labour. At the beginning of July I weighed in at 13 stone 10lb (87 kilos) but, more thrillingly, I discovered that I'd lost 14 centimetres from the circumference of my waist. Jay also did several calliper measurements to ascertain my body fat, which had evidently decreased from 24 per cent to 17 per cent. It was an extremely dramatic turnaround in such a short space of time.

Such was the intensity of my resistance training programme, I had to tweak my diet in order to give my body the right nutritional support. Keen to maintain energy, gain lean muscle and prevent post-workout hunger pangs, I significantly increased my calorific intake. I began to eat four protein-rich meals per day, starting most mornings with a breakfast of two scrambled eggs and a mound of steamed spinach. This would be followed by a lunch, dinner and supper that all contained at least 200 grams of protein. Typically, these three meals would comprise a large portion of fish and meat, of which two would be lean (a chicken breast, a fillet steak or a piece of cod, perhaps) and one would be oily or fatty (perhaps some smoked mackerel or a couple of pork chops). To maintain my carbohydrate intake, I ate as many leafy green vegetables and as much mixed salad as I could manage; I could easily munch my way through a full head of broccoli per day, and two or three bags of baby leaves. In essence I was following a meat and two veg diet, a bit like my mum used to serve up in the 1970s, minus the boiled potatoes and the Bisto gravy.

For me, weight training was transformational – I'd never felt so physically robust – and I only wished I'd started it earlier in my journey. To any middle-aged men reading this who are struggling with their weight, and who are looking to improve their fitness from a standing start, my advice would be this: if you only have time to do two hours a week of training, lift weights. Before you even think about running around the park, or signing up for a spin class, lift weights. Join a good gym, follow the advice from an experienced instructor and approach things slowly and gradually. All I can say is that it worked for me; the increased strength I gained provided an excellent basis for other sports and activities – cycling, swimming, climbing – and I've never looked back.

In addition to pumping iron, I also started pushing pedals. I had first introduced cycling into my fitness regime in 2018, alternating bike rides with my regular walking and jogging sessions. A blend of road bike, touring bike and mountain bike, my Trek hybrid had been bought on a well-intentioned whim a few years previously, but had been left to gather cobwebs in the shed (no surprise there, then). In those days I had neither the confidence nor the inclination to wheel it out in London – heaving my 22-stone frame into the saddle, in a city gridlocked with traffic, sounded like too much of an ordeal for me – and I'd dismissed it as yet another one of my failed fitness fads. When I started to shed weight and get healthy, however, I decided to bring the Trek out of retirement and take it out on the road. Once I'd pumped up the tyres and polished the frame (and pulled on my new padded Lycra shorts), we were both good to go.

It took a few tentative circuits of Vauxhall's cycle lanes to build up my confidence. I had not ridden a bicycle properly for 20 years (I used to pedal my beloved Raleigh Chopper from the Ferndale Estate to Habberley Valley) and I was a little wobbly, in both mind and body. I was determined to master life on two wheels, though. One drizzly afternoon I tackled the incline on Lambeth Bridge – not much of a climb, admittedly – and felt my lungs heaving and my calves burning.

How the hell am I going to get over this? I remember thinking. *C'mon, Tom, dig deep.*

I gripped my handlebars, moved through the gears, reached the mini-summit and headed down toward Black Prince Road. A small victory, but a great feeling.

When I first took up cycling, I primarily saw my hour-long rides as a mode of exercise, and regarded my bike as a piece of outdoor gym equipment. But, as my confidence and competence increased, zipping along the designated cycleways became my favourite mode of transport around the capital. Cycling felt like a way of life, not just an extension of my fitness regime, and I soon found myself opting to travel to Westminster by Trek, not taxi.

One morning Mary Creagh, MP for Wakefield and a

very accomplished cyclist, spotted me tethering my bike to the rack outside the Palace of Westminster.

'Can I just say how fantastic it is to see you cycling, Tom?' she said. 'Hope you get as much out of it as I've done over the years.'

'Cheers, Mary,' I replied. 'I'm absolutely loving it.'

Jeremy Corbyn, himself a keen cyclist, took the opportunity to give me some encouragement, too, as well as some sound advice.

'Never scrimp on your waterproofs,' he said one afternoon following a shadow cabinet meeting. 'Cheap ones always let the rain in. It's worth spending a little extra on something that's really robust.'

'Thanks, Jeremy, I'll bear that in mind,' I said, making a mental note to pay a visit to my local outdoor-fitness emporium.

I also used the bike to motivate and reward myself by applying a kind of rudimentary nudge theory. Each time I hit a weight-loss goal, I'd treat myself to a brand new piece of kit for my bike. In most cases, nothing was of huge monetary value – one week it would be a bottle holder, the next a flashing backlight – but this positive reinforcement really helped me to focus on the task in hand. Perhaps it was the video gamer in me, who'd always loved setting goals, meeting them, and then being rewarded or upgraded for reaching the higher level. My favourite (and perhaps most useful) bike-related purchase was a wire shopping basket that clipped onto my handlebars. This allowed me to stop off at Borough Market or Tesco Vauxhall after work and load up with fresh provisions for that evening's meal. I would always be extra-careful cycling home, however, avoiding any road ramps or potholes that might catapult my free-range eggs and Hass avocados down Kennington Road.

I promised myself a special treat for a symbolic milestone, though.

'If I lose a hundred pounds in weight, I'm buying myself a brand new bike,' I told my brother Dan (a fellow enthusiast) over the phone one evening. While I'd grown very fond of my trusty old Trek, it was quite heavy and clunky, and I fancied something with a little more zip. Not only that, a few communal cycling challenges had caught my eye (there were always plenty of rides going on in London) and I felt that my wheels needed to be a bit more fit for purpose.

In November 2018 my Nokia scales hit that all-important target – 208lb (94 kilos) – but it wasn't until the following spring, when the frost and ice began to clear, that I made my purchase. Prior to that I'd researched all sorts of bikes on the internet, watching countless YouTube videos, trawling through online stockists and wondering whether to opt for a road bike or another hybrid. I also sought advice from a good contact of mine, Andrew Denton, who spearheaded the Outdoor Industries Association, an organisation that encouraged UK citizens, regardless of age or ability, to get outside and get active. Andrew also happened to be a very experienced triathlete who knew a lot about bicycles, and he duly pointed me in the direction of a specialist cycling shop in London. I heeded the advice from an extremely enthusiastic member of staff, and ended up plumping for a sleek-looking, black-framed Focus Izalco road bike, which, as it was a display model, came with a hefty discount. I was ever so slightly worried by the fact that it had cleats – those metal clips that attach cycling shoes to pedals – but I was reassured that I'd get used to them in no time.

'Ha, that's a proper midlife crisis bike,' said my brother, laughing, when I told him about my new purchase.

'Yeah, you're probably right,' I replied. 'The modern-day equivalent of an MGB soft-top…'

I took my new bike out for a few test rides in London, preferring to cycle along wide park avenues rather than congested cycle lanes while I (quite literally) found my feet. Negotiating the cleat mechanism wasn't easy; whenever I came to a halt I had to master the technique of quickly twisting my heel outwards to disengage it from the pedal, in order to avoid crashing down like falling timber. A cyclist pal of mine had joked that I couldn't call myself a proper cyclist until I'd keeled over on my bike at least a dozen times, having failed to release those pesky cleats in a timely manner. By the spring of 2019 I was definitely edging toward that tally.

A few weeks later, I decided to join up with some friends for a camping weekend in Hay-on-Wye, in Herefordshire. One of my favourite towns in the UK, it boasted some awe-inspiring scenery, and was renowned for its glut of second-hand bookshops. I reckoned this mini-break would be the ideal opportunity to give my Izalco a run out along some country lanes – and I really wanted to practise moving through the many gears – so I made plans to take the train from London to Hereford, and to cycle the rest of the twenty-mile route to Hay.

Let's just say I underestimated how difficult and daunting this excursion would be. Even the act of loading the bike onto the train at Paddington was an ordeal. This process was second nature to seasoned cyclists, of course, but as a novice I had no idea which part of the train to use, or how to work the storage racks, and as the departure time loomed I got myself into a bit of a lather. One of the Great Western Railway train managers must have seen me dithering around and came to my rescue, guiding me to the appropriate carriage and demonstrating how to stow the bike safely and securely. GWR, I've since learned, is one of the more cyclist-friendly train operators.

'You're Tom Watson the MP, aren't you?' said the manager, once I'd thanked him for all his help.

'Yes, that's right.' I nodded.

'Thought you were. Didn't recognise you in your Lycra. You used to be quite a big fella, didn't you? No offence, like…'

'None taken.' I smiled.

Three hours later I alighted from the train at Hereford station, gently lowering my bike onto the platform and affixing the panniers containing my belongings. It was an unexpectedly warm spring day – the mid-morning sun was beating down – so I donned my peaked cap and took a few glugs of water before starting my pedal to Hay-on-Wye.

I knew I should have brought that suncream, I thought to myself as I squinted through my cycling glasses.

I had expected the landscape to be quite challenging (there was a lot of up-hill and down-dale), so I roughly estimated my journey time to be around the two-hour mark.

However, about halfway through the journey, and in the middle of nowhere, I got horribly lost. Like an idiot, I'd left my handlebar phone holster at home, so had been unable to track the route as I'd cycled and had clearly taken a wrong turn. The signs for Hay-on-Wye had petered out, and there was neither a house nor a human in sight. When I stopped at a lay-by and fished my phone from my pannier, I discovered there was no signal and, without anything as sensible as a backup map in my bag, I realised I was on my own.

Things became even worse. As my body flagged, and my water dwindled, I found myself faced with a steep, snaking hill, probably amounting to a 1:4 gradient. It was the kind of zigzag slope that experienced cyclists tackled with consummate ease, but that biking beginners viewed with sheer panic. Yet, that said, I was bloody well determined not to get out of the saddle and walk it. I had bought this bike as a vehicle, not a prop.

C'mon, Tom, give it all you've got... I said to myself. *Just imagine you're Bradley Wiggins climbing the Alpe d'Huez...*

About halfway up the incline, as my energy finally began to wane, a huge tractor suddenly roared past me, straddling the white lines in the road and spluttering diesel fumes in its wake. Taken by surprise, I instantly stopped pedalling and swerved out of the way to avoid the tractor. I failed to take my feet 'n' cleats out of the pedals, though, and tumbled into a verge of stinging nettles, turning the Herefordshire air blue as I did so (Sir Bradley would have done the same, I reckoned). I slowly dragged myself up and dusted myself off, but then noticed a trickle of blood dripping down my leg where I'd gashed it on a rock.

Tom, you fucking idiot...

After cleaning up the wound with the last dregs of my water bottle, I continued the half-mile trek up the hill (albeit on foot) and, once I'd reached the summit, I clambered gingerly back into the saddle. The road was riven with boneshaking craters and potholes but, as I freewheeled to the bottom – *hallelujah* – I finally spotted a sign for Hay-on-Wye.

An hour later I turned up at the campsite with a bloodied leg, a sunburnt forehead and a mouth as dry as the Serengeti. Weirdly, though, I'd never felt so exhilarated. Though my Tour de Hereford hadn't exactly gone to plan, I'd completed my first ever long(ish)-distance countryside cycle. It was something that, three years previously, I'd never have thought possible.

When I returned to London, still smarting from the nettle stings, I thought it might be wise to attend a Bikeability course. A cycling training programme – a modern-day version of the old Cycling Proficiency Test, in many respects – it teaches practical skills to participants in order to increase their confidence on the road. As someone who had returned to cycling later in life I found it immensely useful, and I learned a heck of a lot from the Bikeability instructors, Gavin and Michael. They noticed that I rode far too close to the kerb, for instance – for my own safety, I needed to properly survey my road space – and I was nowhere near decisive enough when I turned left or right at junctions. Taking these observations on board, and understanding my rights on the road, made a huge difference to my day-to-day cycling. After three lessons I had the confidence to cycle along Regent Street and around the roundabouts of Piccadilly and Trafalgar Square, something that had always terrified me in the past.

Attending the Bikeability course prompted me to think more deeply about cycling policy and culture. I read a marvellous book called *Bike Nation: How Cycling Can Save the World* by Peter Walker, which explored the different attitudes to cycling on highways across the globe and investigated the problems that cyclists faced, from aggressive truck drivers to obstructive town planners. I also started to speak at various cycling-related events, including some organised by Labour Cycles, a lobby group campaigning for 'social justice on our roads and active travel for all'. During those meetings I called for increased investment into cycling infrastructure – including a fundamental change in UK road design, and the reallocation of highway space for cycle lanes – and I challenged workplaces to offer more bike-friendly facilities, from secure storage lockers to staff shower blocks.

I also talked about the role that cycling could play in reversing health inequalities and reducing carbon emissions, and how local, regional and national government had a duty to make it safer, easier and more enjoyable for people to get into the saddle and become more active. 'Stealth-health,' I called it: improving your fitness while at the same time having fun, whether that meant reaching the summit of Lambeth Bridge, or freewheeling down a Herefordshire hillside.

CHAPTER SEVEN

Tackling Big Sugar

When I woke up from a lifetime of abusing my body with a poor diet, I felt a little like Jim Carrey's character at the end of *The Truman Show*. When his boat struck the metal dome masquerading as a skyline, I was reminded of my own sense of dismay and disillusion after realising that, for decades, I'd effectively been duped. Truman, like me, came to learn that everything he'd been encouraged and programmed to presume was natural was in fact fabricated, in order to trap and exploit him.

For me, the boat scene was the perfect metaphor for how the food industry has synthetically reshaped what we eat in order to trap and exploit us. They tell us that we choose what we eat and how we feed ourselves, even as they knowingly manipulate us into becoming addicted to an unnatural and unhealthy diet. We are all Trumans, living in a world that has been carefully constructed by industry. And that architecture, that world remade in the interests of massive industrial corporations, is making us fat.

Key to comprehending these food 'choices' is the understanding that human beings do not need sugar. Seriously. It is not a case of 'we need to eat and drink less sugar'; it's a case of not needing to eat sugar at all. Way back in 1972, the renowned physiologist and nutritionist John

Yudkin argued this case in his groundbreaking book, *Pure, White and Deadly*:

'First, there is no physiological requirement for sugar,' he wrote. 'All human nutritional needs can be met without having to take a single spoon of white or brown or raw sugar, on its own or in any food or drink. Secondly, if only a small fraction of what is already known about the effects of sugar were to be revealed in relation to any other material used as a food additive, that material would promptly be banned.'

When you realise this, you can't help but see that the food industry – driven by so-called 'Big Sugar' corporations – has fundamentally reformed the basic assumptions that underpin our relationship with food, diet and nutrition. Once you accept that sugar is not a nutritionally necessary part of any foodstuff, it is hard not to feel real anger at the absurdities of manufacturers producing 'lower-sugar' versions of their products (which needn't have had sugar added in the first place). Our taste buds and our expectations have been re-engineered to make us pliant addicts to a product that human beings don't need, and which has potentially deadly consequences, but which we have been trained to desire and expect in every mouthful.

As Christof, the control-freak director in *The Truman Show*, says: 'We accept the reality of the world with which we are presented. It's as simple as that.'

These things start in childhood. What our kids learn about food and about eating – what is often taught as 'normal'

– shapes their habits and their choices throughout their life. When I was a kid, around the time that Western society began its transition from home-made fare to factory-produced food, we didn't unduly worry about sugar content. Indeed, mass-produced cereal was considered the ideal breakfast option in the 1970s – *'They're grrreat!'* growled Tony the Tiger in the Kellogg's TV adverts – and I'd shovel down two or three bowls of Frosties in one sitting, savouring every mouthful of those sweet 'n' crunchy flakes. My brekkie would be accompanied by a glass of 'fresh' concentrated orange juice, which, in those days, was the height of sophistication since it was a step up from luminous orange squash. My siblings and I had got through three or four bottles of squash a week – we'd often guzzled it undiluted – until it was taken off supermarket shelves due to it containing the synthetic colouring E102 (tartrazine), which was found to cause hyperactivity in children. I seem to remember the scandal being reported by Esther Rantzen on her consumer show, *That's Life!*

Concentrated orange juice, however, was still deemed a much healthier option.

'Anyone for a top-up?' Mom would ask, brandishing a carton. 'Full of vitamin C, it says here…'

'Thanks, Mom,' I'd say, as she filled up my glass.

As we approached our teens, however, it became common knowledge that sugary cereals actually weren't the best way to start the day, and had a detrimental effect on your dietary and dental health. My mum decided instead to embrace the *en vogue* continental breakfast, and began filling our bread bin with croissants, pain au chocolat and French baguettes. I often preferred a 'proper' loaf, though – white Mother's Pride in a waxed wrapper, bought from Vera's local shop on Hurcott Road – and would fix myself three or four slices of toast and butter before school. Sometimes I'd slather on a thick layer of strawberry jam, blissfully unaware that, within a few years, my sweet tooth would develop into a full-blown sugar addiction.

In the 1980s, convenience food was king. Processed meals that you warmed up in the oven (usually served with McCain's Oven Chips) were commonplace in the Watson household, and Indian or Chinese takeaways became regular weekend treats. As a boy, I distinctly remember the day that Mom took delivery of our first ever chest freezer. She had watched a news report on *Nationwide* about families who'd saved a fortune by bulk-buying from specialist frozen food centres, and there was no way she was going to miss out.

'I'm off to Comet... they've got a sale on,' she said one Saturday morning, and a week later our brand new appliance arrived, ready to be plugged in and stocked up with Ross Quarter-Pounders, Findus Crispy Pancakes and a multicoloured selection of ice creams and lollipops. Meg, Dan and I relished this treasure trove of frozen goodies, in particular the Bird's Eye Arctic Rolls. We thought these ice cream 'n' sponge desserts were a taste sensation, so much so that we went to the ridiculous lengths of measuring each portion with a ruler to ensure equal slices.

Plenty more time-saving gadgets appeared in the

kitchen, too (or 'mod cons' as we called them), including a newfangled Breville toastie maker. Such was Mom's resourcefulness, she'd bag up left-over sandwiches from family gatherings, put them in her handbag and freeze them at home, to reheat them in the Breville a few days later.

We didn't appreciate the damage that convenience food was doing to us – there was no food education in this respect, and very little in the way of public health guidelines – and my parents would have been horrified had they realised the long-term effects these products were having on their offspring's health. And besides, back in the 1970s, fake food was being sold to working-class people as liberation. Why slave away in the kitchen making tea for the family when you could throw in some fish fingers and oven chips and keep everyone happy, with hardly any fuss? We wolfed down mountains of chemically reconstructed, additive-stuffed synthetic imitations of actual food. We drank lakes of sugar that burst with bubbles and never quite quenched our thirst (I glugged bottle after bottle of dandelion and burdock, a treacly concoction distributed by our local 'pop man'). And we got fat.

But we didn't blame the food that we ate or the fizz that we drank. No, we blamed ourselves. Because the industry that had spent billions refining that food to make it ever more convenient, and ever more addictive, was cleverer than us. They had already taught ordinary people that the fault was not the food, the fault was the people *eating* the food. So, as childhood obesity increased, a clamour went up – in the media, from think-tanks and from organisations funded by the sugar industry – that Western kids were getting porky because they didn't do enough exercise. That argument, conceived in (and promoted by) the food-factory owners, came to dominate any discussion of this massive public health crisis. It served as a distraction. It bought a lot of people off. It kept us eating, and it taught us to loathe ourselves and others for lacking the get-up-and-go of previous 'more active' generations.

If you have to admire one thing about the industrialists who control what we eat, then it has to be their chutzpah. You or I would be compelled to act if we discovered that the product we made and sold was harming children. We would reduce the sugar and the additives that we knew were turning ordinary members of the public into addicts. We would warn people to stop treating what was once a convenient snack as a staple of their diet. We would halt the production lines that churned out food that we knew was giving individuals diabetes and was clogging their arteries. Not these fellas, though. They did none of that. Determined to thwart any efforts to modify their products to reduce their harmful nature, they instead re-engineered public discourse and public policy. Like I say, you can't accuse the food industry of lacking ambition or cunning. Just basic morality.

Some people will say that this is over-egging the pudding a little. Surely these firms didn't really know the harm that they were doing? And there's nothing wrong with telling people to get off their sofa and start exercising, is there? Let's take each of these in turn.

Did the food industry know what it was doing? Absolutely it did. As I began to dig my way out of my obesity I read everything I could get my hands on about the history of the food business. I wanted to understand how we'd arrived at where we are today. I wanted to know why I felt like Truman, discovering that what I'd believed to be normal had in fact been fabricated in order to exploit me.

One of the books that really transformed my understanding of the food industry and its machinations was *Salt, Sugar, Fat: How the Food Giants Hooked Us* by Michael Moss, a Pulitzer Prize-winning US journalist. No one who read even the introduction to that book would have dared plead ignorance in defence of Big Food Inc. It includes the following:

> Some of the largest companies are now using brain scans to study how we react neurologically to certain foods, especially to sugar. They've discovered that the brain lights up for sugar the same way it does for cocaine, and this knowledge is useful, not only in formulating foods. The world's biggest ice cream maker, Unilever, for instance, parlayed its brain research into a brilliant marketing campaign that sells the eating of ice cream as a way to make ourselves happy.

Moss, a brilliant investigative reporter, unearthed some fascinating nuggets of information. He recounted an extraordinary (and clandestine) meeting in 1999 that convened the MDs and CEOs of America's largest food corporations. Representatives of Kraft were in attendance, as were others from Tate & Lyle, Nestlé and General Mills. And one of their own – a brave soul named Michael Mudd, a Kraft vice president – stood up before them and laid out exactly the harm that they, collectively, were doing to public health. He showed them the evidence, he told it straight and he pleaded with them to take action to reduce the poison in their products, and to review the marketing strategies they employed. They said no.

My quest for knowledge led me to the work of another campaigning author. The highly respected American academic, Dr Marion Nestle, had spent a lifetime researching nutritional science and public health in order to understand the impact of diet upon us all. In her book, *Soda Politics: Taking on Big Soda (And Winning)*, Dr Nestle (a confusing surname for an intrepid opponent of Big Sugar, I'll grant you) detailed how companies like Coca-Cola and PepsiCo presented two faces to the world. They spent billions marketing directly to children and young people, to normalise the consumption of their highly dangerous, industrialised products. At the same time, they generously gifted money to charities and bodies that were tasked with tackling childhood obesity, a problem for which they were at least partially responsible, and which they and their products exacerbated every day.

Dr Nestle outlined how these companies had poured money into anti-regulation lobbying, estimating that Coca-

Cola alone had sanctioned a global spend of $100 million in order to oppose sugar legislation. Her findings certainly ruffled some feathers. In fact, the octogenarian was considered so dangerous to American corporate interests (despite having once worked for President Reagan) that she was mentioned in the Wikileaks dump of diplomatic cables in 2016.

I was truly privileged to meet Dr Nestle in person in July 2019, when she and I got together in my Westminster office, where the bookshelves contained a number of her titles. Indeed, having read so many of her studies, I felt like I was meeting a hero. We discussed the huge global network of lobby interests, stacked against those who were raising increasing concerns about the balance of refined sugar in our daily diets.

'Good luck in your battles to come, Tom,' she said at the end of our conversation, with great understatement.

'I won't let you down,' I replied.

Although Michael Mudd's plan for the rehabilitation and redemption of his industry was largely rebuffed by his peers, they did adopt one of his recommendations: the promotion of exercise. While some people lauded the food corporations for putting so much effort (and so much money) into encouraging fitness and activity, others were far more cynical, viewing it as a conniving, albeit clever move. No sane or responsible person was going to stand up and declare that kids should exercise less, that inactivity was a good thing, or that sitting in front of the telly all day was a healthy alternative to a kickabout in the park.

Exercise, of course, played a massive role in my own recovery. Aged 50, I'd struggled to get up a flight of stairs to reach my office, yet aged 52, I was lifting weights and riding a bike. I have never dismissed the importance of keeping yourself fit, active and mobile, but the truth of the matter is that exercise alone cannot solve the obesity crisis. The adage that you can 'eat what you like, so long as you exercise' is a pernicious lie.

What we now know is that, while preaching active lifestyles as the answer to the problem, these companies are manufacturing food that is so drenched in sugar and additives that it makes it harder – psychologically and physiologically – to get into a routine of regular exercise. And that's before we even get to the fact that, in order to burn off the calories found in one can of Coca-Cola, you'd have to walk five miles (eight kilometres) or run for fifty minutes. In 2016, the average UK teenager was drinking 234 cans of fizzy pop a year. That would take 1,170 miles (1,883 kilometres) of walking to burn off, or more than three miles (five kilometres) per day; all that just to neutralise the impact of one product on our kids' lives. When you factor in the sugar and calorie impact of the whole gamut of processed foodstuffs that our children are consuming on a daily basis, you'd need to chain your offspring to a treadmill if you seriously believed that exercise could be the whole answer.

That is why we need to break the links that these 'Big

Sugar' brands have built with sports teams and bodies in the UK. When Coca-Cola sponsors the Premier League or Müller funds British Athletics, they aren't just innocently laundering their profits through a good cause. They are associating their products with exercise, effectively teaching young people that, after a runaround, it's safe and healthy to 'treat' yourself to a can of fizzy pop or a sugar-laden yoghurt. It isn't. I think one of the key culprits in this enormous rise in obesity and diabetes is the sugar industry and, in the same way that we don't allow tobacco companies to sponsor sports, we need to get on with banning Big Sugar from promoting itself via brand relationships. Frankly, the Premier League (which can certainly afford to take the financial hit) should be taking action itself rather than waiting for government to force its hand.

'What images come to mind when you think about Coca-Cola?' I asked in a speech in early 2019.

'Do you think about young healthy people engaging in sports and having fun together? Or do you think about overweight diabetes patients lying in a hospital bed? Drinking lots of Coca-Cola will not make you young, will not make you healthy, will not make you athletic; rather it increases your chances of suffering from obesity and diabetes.

'Yet, for decades, Coca-Cola has invested billions of dollars in linking itself to youth, health and sports, and billions of humans believe in this linkage.'

Not only is it ridiculous to allow a fizzy pop manufacturer to associate itself with the beautiful game, it is also dangerous.

It is a sobering statistic that children in the UK aged

four to ten are now estimated to consume 5,500 cubes of sugar per year; that's about 3.5 stone (22 kilos) worth of the sweet stuff, or the weight of an average three-year-old. Little wonder, then, that we have the worst childhood obesity rates in Western Europe, and that more children than ever are being admitted to hospital with rotten teeth. And it was against this backdrop that, in 2019, I lent my support to the 'Fizz Free February' initiative. Established by Southwark Council the previous year, it encouraged local residents to give up fizzy drinks for a whole month. Designed to address health concerns, Fizz Free February also fought back against corporations that profited from excessive sugar consumption. It attracted some significant endorsements along the way, too.

'Prevention matters to us, because we see the damage fizzy drinks do every day,' commented Mick Armstrong, Chair of the British Dental Association, who fully backed the campaign.

'The idea behind Fizz Free February couldn't be simpler: simply encourage families to take a few weeks out from reaching for a can of pop,' he added. 'This idea may have started small over in Southwark, but we're proud to help this campaign go national.'

I encouraged many other Labour authorities to get on board (including my own, Sandwell in the West Midlands, with great leadership from Councillor Elaine Costigan) and enlisted the help of health secretary Matt Hancock and his shadow, my colleague Jonathan Ashworth. Hugh Fearnley-Whittingstall – the feted cook and food writer – was also happy to associate himself with the scheme. Like me, Hugh had successfully lost weight by eradicating sugar from his diet and was a long-time critic of the sugar industry, a subject he'd explored in his excellent BBC series, *Britain's Fat Fight*.

A Fizz Free February information pack, which raised awareness of sugar-related obesity, was distributed to a variety of business and educational locations. I learned of one participating school that asked its students to hand in any cans of pop at registration, only allowing them to be collected at home time. The benefits of drinking water were promoted throughout the day, and pupils were given the chance to earn rewards points for bringing reusable water bottles to school.

During that particular month, I remember having a frank and honest conversation with my 11-year-old daughter about her sugary drink intake. I had always tried to encourage my kids to restrict their consumption of sweet things, although I'd stopped short of imposing an outright ban.

'Did you know, Saoirse,' I said, 'that your favourite coffee chain sells a banana milkshake that contains the equivalent of *thirty-nine* teaspoons of sugar? That's the equivalent of nearly fifteen KitKats in one glass.'

'Oh, right...' She shrugged. 'That doesn't sound good.'

A few days later I took Saoirse for a bite to eat at that same coffee emporium, and asked her what she fancied to drink.

'I'd like one of those banana milkshakes please,' she said, with a mischievous glint in her eye.

It was a telling moment, and taught me a couple of things. Firstly, that my daughter was developing a decidedly rebellious streak and a wicked sense of humour. And secondly, when it came to the war on sugar, I'd always have a battle on my hands, whether as a parent or a politician.

The 'active lifestyles' line is not the only lobbying and communications tool that the food industry has deployed to shield themselves from blame. There are plenty of others. They label efforts to increase the prices of their unhealthiest products as 'sin taxes'. They insinuate that there's nothing wrong with people wanting to treat themselves, and that anyone denying them this pleasure is promoting a 'nanny state'. They claim that attacks on convenience foods are the result of classist, snobbish interference in working-class lifestyles, as though it's somehow inherent in certain cultures to gravitate toward a harmful diet.

What all of these suppositions have in common is that they place the burden of responsibility solely on the individual. It is *your* choice what to eat and to drink, and it is *your* fault if you choose poorly. But it's not. I was a sugar addict because my supply chain of food was malfunctioning; it didn't give me the options I needed to get well. And now that I am well, and am off sugar, I realise that people don't often have easily digestible information at their disposal. The decisions I was forced to make were artificial, and were made within an architecture designed to suit Big Sugar.

They took place in a world that food corporations carefully re-engineered in order to push me in a particular direction.

Indeed, I remember sweating for an hour on a static bike in a Victoria gym in the mid-1990s – another of my failed fitness attempts – only to undo all the effort with a can of Coke from the reception vending machine.

These firms hide sugar in foods they call healthy. They market to you from the moment you are born to cultivate your sweet tooth. They spend billions refining their products and their packaging to keep you coming back. They reframe our choices by creating 'healthier' versions of their dangerous products so that you can feel somewhat virtuous when you opt for just 'bad' over 'very bad'. And they tell you not to worry too much because you can always go jogging to work it all off.

Just as Truman discovered that his life was carefully constructed around him – creating the illusion of free will, and presenting an alternative to reality – we also operate under the pretence of self-will, while in truth we are engineered toward more synthesised food and less wholesome produce.

In *Salt, Sugar, Fat*, Michael Moss explained how the line between nutritional science and product development had been blurred and manipulated by the food industry. This was best exemplified by the 'bliss point' – the perfect balance of sugar, fat and salt within a product to 'send consumers over the moon' – for which scientists and researchers in the pay of Big Sugar were searching. They knew that the tipping point between a tasty product and an addictive one was found at this juncture, and they refined and redesigned until they manufactured it.

This was a science, yes. But it was more akin to *Breaking Bad*'s Walter White cooking meth in his lab than to public-spirited professionals trying to work out what was actually good for us. Moss was right to describe sugar as the 'methamphetamine of processed food ingredients'. The food industry has been spending billions disfiguring the scientific landscape by focusing research not on how we can feed ourselves well, but on how we can make non-nutritional foods more addictive. This has been one very powerful way in which Big Sugar has re-engineered our choices.

It is a massive public policy issue that needs to be seriously addressed. I am determined that my children should grow up in a society in which their ability to live healthy lives doesn't depend solely on their sheer wilfulness. It is the job of government to protect people from those who would wield power over them. However, that power is often hidden, and sometimes it offends our sense of ourselves as free-thinking individuals to concede that we are being controlled. But government's job is to step in, to step up and to push back against those who seek to manipulate us to our own detriment. That is my core philosophy. And it applies to Big Food as much as it does to unscrupulous bankers, exploitative bosses and power-hungry media barons.

So what do we have to do? We have to revolutionise our food industry so that it serves the many, not the few. And we need to start with sugar. I have been left gobsmacked by the sugar industry's arrogance and sense of entitlement. These firms are so used to being left to their own devices, without much in the way of scrutiny or accountability, that they seem genuinely affronted by calls for greater transparency and more forceful regulation. They behave as though they have a divine right to peddle their product no matter the harm that it causes. This attitude, and this behaviour, has to change.

The truth is that these businesses profit from other people's misery. They have a vested and direct financial interest in adding their product, in ever more inventive ways, to more and more of our food. They conspire with manufacturers and retailers to hide the sugar that they add to products, so that consumers find it harder to choose healthier alternatives. They market directly to very young children in the knowledge that developing a sweet palate at an early age predisposes children to eat more and more sugar as they get older, and makes it harder for them to live well. We aggressively tax tobacco, alcohol and petrol not just to raise revenue, but also to acknowledge the harm that these products do, and to seek to change consumer perception by nudging people toward behaviour that is better for them and for the world. We need to do the same with sugar.

In 2018 the UK introduced a small, limited levy of between 18p and 24p per litre on soft drinks that contain more than five grams of sugar per 100 millilitres. It was a modest measure, designed to rein in the makers of the fizzy pop that rots our kids' teeth and can make them fat. To me, the success of the Soft Drinks Industry Levy – otherwise known as the sugar tax – was an illustration that government can and should intervene if the food and drink industry won't do it themselves.

The industry's response in the run-up to the levy being imposed was nothing short of hysterical. The big drinks companies fought the sugar tax tooth and nail, saying that it wouldn't work, and that it would be impossible to alter the composition of their products. Industry representatives claimed that taxing super-sugary drinks would lead to job losses and would damage business, while their allies and lobbyists in Westminster think-tanks argued that this represented some existential assault on consumer freedom.

These days, the companies hide behind false-flag campaign groups. You only have to take a look at the @AgainstSugarTax account on Twitter. I have no idea who funds this campaign, but it instigates the trolling of propaganda that only helps Coca-Cola and Kellogg's to defend the status quo.

Once the tax was introduced, however, almost overnight the manufacturers of Ribena — Suntory — cut the blackcurrant drink's sugar content by half in order to avoid a levy-related price rise. Since then, more than half of all sweet beverages have been reformulated. It has been a stunning public health success. Some contrarians, however, still regard the levy as a failure because it only raised half as much cash for the exchequer as initially predicted. But accruing money was not the reason for the tax in the first place; it was introduced to change behaviour. And it did so, in a fascinating and encouraging way. It forced Big Sugar to change its approach rather than placing the burden of choice on consumers themselves. It altered the business model and it intervened upstream.

To a certain sort of politician, this development was genuinely horrifying. It was one thing to occasionally interfere with personal freedom, but the liberty of the corporation was sacrosanct. From my perspective, however, the effectiveness of the sugar tax was a beacon of hope within our obesity crisis, as it forced a small section of the food industry to change their behaviour in the interests of public health.

Perhaps it's now time to impose the levy on other drinks, like milkshakes – as the Department for Health has recommended – and to explore how we can also apply it to food, in order to force a change in formulation and ingredients. I should emphasise, however, that this is not about making ordinary people pay more for the food they need. It is about forcing a change, at source, so that members of the public can eat well without having hidden sugar forced down their throats. It is poorer individuals in society who are most vulnerable to obesity, and to the conditions and illnesses that this can lead to. Don't let cynical politicians and industrialists take these people's names in vain when opposing sensible measures like the sugar tax. You do poor people no favours when you keep the price of bad food low.

We also need to tackle the skewing of the science by corporate billions, as identified by Michael Moss and Marion Nestle. Our understanding of nutrition is lagging behind where it should be because, for decades, Big Sugar and the food industry have focused resources and attention on making food more addictive, not making it more nutritious. A new levy, requesting food companies to hand over a proportion of their research and development budget to an independent nutritional research council, should be introduced. The council would then distribute these funds — matched, maybe, by government money — in order to look into proposals on a system of merit, guided by public good. In this way we could start to rebalance the focus of food and nutrition research, giving us a more level playing field in the battle for Britain's bellies.

What I've learned over the years is that the food labelling system in the UK is broken, particularly in relation to sugar. Having been hoodwinked by misleading packaging myself, I've done my utmost to publicly highlight the dangers of hidden sugars in our food. Even if you forgo the obvious culprits — sweets, cakes and biscuits — you're still being exposed to huge amounts in products where you'd perhaps least expect it, such as cereals, soups and sauces. Indeed, I've found that everything from pizzas to sandwiches, and from 'energy' bars to 'health' drinks, contains more sugar than you'd ever imagine. All too often, where foods are labelled 'low-fat' (think yoghurts, ice cream or salad dressings), extra sugar has been added to make up for the loss of taste. Food production is all based on a sugar economy. Even trying to avoid sugar is difficult.

Dr Robert Lustig addressed this in his seminal book, *Fat Chance: The Hidden Truth about Sugar, Obesity and Disease*:

By using different forms of sugar in any given product, the food industry can add many different sugars to one product. The grams don't change, but the order on the label does. The food industry has over forty other names for sugar in an effort to hide it on the label, but a discerning eye can often spot them.

He then cited the various names that are used on food labels to describe sugar, including fructose, dextrose and maltodextrin, as well as the deceptively wholesome-sounding barley malt, agave nectar and blackstrap molasses. The sugar content is hidden in plain sight behind complicated names; to be a health-conscious shopper these days, it seems you need a GCSE in biology to decipher the nutritional information.

In November 2018 I penned an article for the *Daily Mail* (the newspaper resumed contact with me following editor Paul Dacre's departure) in which I exposed the misleading labels found on brands in our high-street supermarkets. I discovered high-sugar juice drinks (being heralded as 'one of your five-a-day') that were made 'partially from concentrate'. The sugar content was not immediately obvious, but the mandatory labelling elsewhere on the 200ml carton confirmed there was 10.5g sugar per 100ml. By including just one such drink in their child's lunchbox, parents would be giving them 21g of sugar, three grams shy of the daily recommended intake of sugar for a seven-to-ten-year-old. As for baby rusks – a staple of infant diets for generations, and once marketed as teething aids – I found that sugar was often the main ingredient after flour. Even the reduced-sugar varieties contained 3.4g per rusk, meaning that an older child who consumed three or four per day could easily hit half their recommended sugar intake.

'Is it any wonder that kids of eight years old are being diagnosed with type 2 diabetes?' I said to Barbara Hearn, a member of my team who'd assisted me with the research.

'It's shocking,' she replied, as we wandered down a central London supermarket aisle. 'All these hidden sugars in food meant for kids. Cereals. Pizza. Even sausages, for goodness sake. Retailers and manufacturers need to be more responsible. We can't just blame parents.'

Barbara and I came across scores of products aimed at youngsters that had little or no nutritional value, food that would arguably make them unwell. It was a hugely dispiriting experience.

Some food for grown-ups was just as bad. In one supermarket I came across a ham and cheese sandwich that contained 15.1g of sugar (or four teaspoons, half the recommended daily allowance). Throw in a packet of crisps and a can of pop to qualify for the discounted 'meal deal', and you'd be over your daily sugar limit in one sitting. In another high-street food store, I found countless chilled chicken products containing honey, dextrose or molasses.

The manufacturers, no doubt, would argue that these additional ingredients are essential as a preservative, or for flavour, but I don't buy it. Foods that don't normally contain sugar shouldn't have it added, and consumers buying a piece of chicken shouldn't expect it to be laden with the stuff. It is thoroughly disingenuous. Maple-roasted, honey-basted, sweet chilli… it's all sugar. Pure and simple.

The way we market food, especially to young consumers, has to undergo radical change, too. The people who sell us our food have immense power over what we end up eating, and we need to tackle the way in which these retailers influence our choices, whether it's McDonald's running Monopoly-themed promotions that encourage kids to supersize their already deeply unhealthy meal, or supermarkets running BOGOF offers on meals saturated with fat and sugar. A particularly insidious example is Coca-Cola's Christmas truck tour, which targets children in various UK towns and cities by handing out free cans from red lorries festooned with fairy lights. In 2018 it was forced to scale back its schedule following opposition from local authorities and public health organisations, all rightly concerned that this flagrant marketing stunt had no benefit to their communities, many of which had significant problems with obesity and tooth decay. I shared their indignation and fired off an angry letter to Coca-Cola Great Britain, stating in no uncertain terms that this festive sampling of sugary drinks was wholly unacceptable.

I had the world of advertising in my sights, too, and in January 2019 delivered a speech to its trade body, the Advertising Association, calling on the industry to stop using cartoon characters on cereal packets to promote sugary products to children. I may not have been the most popular person in the conference hall that morning, but some home truths needed telling.

'We face a public health crisis in the UK, and one of the main causes is refined sugar in our foods and drinks,' I said. 'The results are horrific: 26,000 children hospitalised with rotten teeth. The worst obesity rates in Western Europe. And the catastrophe of type 2 diabetes, taking lives and costing the NHS £10 billion a year. I'm making it my political mission to change this.'

I then projected up some images of various Kellogg's cereal packets, complete with garish colours and grinning characters: Tony the Tiger, the Honey Monster, the Coco Pops monkey.

'Before anyone tells me this is packaging and not advertising, let me tell you what they are: they are advertising billboards on tabletops aimed at tiny tots. And, because of that, they should be included in the self-regulatory arrangements for the industry.

'These products are packed full of sugar, with little nutritional value. Even if a child had the recommended portion of Frosties, they'd be eating more than half their daily allowance of sugar before they've even got to school. And if they ate a bowl the size of the one that's depicted on the front of the pack, they'd be exceeding their daily sugar allowance in one sitting. For children under ten, cereal is their single biggest source of free sugar intake. When we have a third of children leaving primary school overweight or obese, when teenage diabetes is rising by seventy per cent, we've got to ask ourselves is this still acceptable? I don't think it is.

'The unpalatable truth for the Advertising Association, which represents the interests of the industry to government, is that some sectors of the advertising industry have played a part in getting us here. Advertising has contributed to making us a nation overweight, unhealthy and addicted to sugar, and the industry has got to play a part in getting us out of this mess. So when it comes to high-sugar products like Coco Pops, my argument to you today is: get that monkey off our packs. I want you to find a way to help us get healthier. Get cartoon characters off adverts for high-sugar foods. Help us kick our sugar habit.

'Everywhere our citizens look, on TV, online, on buses, on billboards, they are surrounded by adverts for foods laced with sugar. Those ads work. They've sold us the idea that breakfast means a bowl of sugary cereal. They've sold us the thought that thirst can only be truly quenched by a sugary, fizzy drink. So, today, I want you to think deeply about how advertising could help transform the lives of Britain's 3.4 million identified type 2 diabetics. How changes in your industry could contribute to stopping kids leaving school obese. How we can get two million type 2 diabetics off their meds. How we can save the NHS ten per cent of its budget.'

The harsh fact is that food packaging laws allow manufacturers to be unacceptably unclear about how much sugar a product contains. A claim such as 'one of your five-a-day' can convince a consumer that the product is healthy, and can distract from the heaps of sugar it actually contains. It doesn't seem right that we allow the sale of 'child-friendly' products with bright colours and jolly illustrations when their contents are close to the recommended daily sugar limit for youngsters. It is not fair to parents or to children.

If we are serious about dealing with our obesity and diabetes epidemics, we've got to get a grip on this issue. At the moment it's like the Wild West. Local trading standards are supposed to have an overview on packaging, but what can they do against a food giant? TV food advertisements are regulated by the Advertising Standards Authority, while nutrition and allergen labelling is monitored by the Food Standards Agency. Too many products fall through the gap and instead of truthful packaging, we are getting packets of lies. Today, when we are reminded of the terrible consequences of diabetes on our personal and national health, we must resolve to do something about it. With all the hidden sugar, conflicting health advice, ultra-processed food and misleading labels, people who want to get healthy barely have a chance.

We can't afford to continue as we are. The scale of the public health crisis that already costs our NHS £10 billion a year is clear. I don't want to live in a society in which people get ill from the food they eat, and then have to fight like hell to regain their health. I don't want my children and grandchildren to go through what I and millions of other people have. These future generations will suffer greatly if we fail to get a grip.

But there are things that my colleagues and I can do to help remedy this. Tackling Big Sugar and fighting the obesity crisis is a massive issue for public policy, and there comes a time when politicians of all sides must join forces to enact change. We need to tackle the global sugar giants who peddle poisons to our children. We need to crack down on junk food adverts on TV and on the high street. We need to ban firms from using children's characters on food packaging if the contents within are loaded with sugar. We need to make laws – like the sugar tax – to enforce change where the industry has palpably failed to show any responsibility. We need to arrive at the point where it's socially unacceptable to drink sugar in pop, where it's considered a little bit dirty and unsavoury. I would like us to replicate what has happened with tobacco, whereby smokers are made to feel shameful and guilty, with products hidden behind screens or under counters. We need to stop tolerating those brands which seek to rake in billions at the expense of our nation's health, and we need to shame them into changing ingredients and clarifying labels.

Encouragingly, however, I do think there is an increasing number of people who are quitting sugar for health reasons (particularly millennials, I reckon, who seem to be relatively food-savvy) and the more that do, the more their cautionary tales and personal testimonies will be heard. If we are to have any hope of forging a healthier society, though, we cannot depend on individuals all enjoying their own epiphany before it's too late. We need to tear down the walls that Big Sugar has built to protect its products and its profits.

Finally, nutritionists may argue about the merits of various diets, but they nearly all agree on two fundamental principles: firstly, that the one-size-fits-all approach no longer works and, secondly, that sugar is extremely bad for you. The sooner we all wise up to this, the sooner we can start building a better, healthier, more nutritious world for everyone.

CHAPTER EIGHT

Remission for All

By 2025 it is estimated that there will be five million people in the UK – nearly five times the population of Birmingham – with a diagnosis of diabetes. Five million of us living with this debilitating disease, searching for answers and seeking a healthier life. The cost to the individual is well known, as is the price paid by society. The National Health Service ploughs £10 billion a year into the treatment of diabetes and that outlay will only rise as the number of sufferers grows.

£10 billion. More than the entire policing budget for England and Wales. Most of that money is spent on treating diabetes-related complications: the increased risk of dementia, sight loss and kidney disease, for example, not forgetting the circulatory problems that can lead to nerve damage and amputation. However, if we can arrest the development of diabetes, we will be able to massively improve people's lives and prevent the next generation from getting sick like we did. And, while lifting millions of people out of the misery and hopelessness of a diabetes diagnosis, we can save the taxpayer a fortune. The good news is that we can stem the flow. The solution is surprisingly simple and shockingly straightforward. I call it Remission for All. And I want it to become a reality in the UK.

Look at it this way. If five million people in our country

contracted leprosy – a truly horrendous condition that rots your body from the outside in – we'd hear an awful lot about it. Legions of people losing their lives and limbs to this disease would prompt a national crisis. There would be urgent questions tabled in parliament, our government would face a public outcry and citizens wouldn't be able to move for action plans and emergency investment. Yet with diabetes – a condition that rots from the inside out – nobody seems to lift a finger. The number of patients rises, and more of us suffer and die, but the response from the corridors of power is slow, muted and lacking in any sense of urgency. And it's not as if we're waiting on some miracle cure or some billion-pound research to fix this, either. Type 2 diabetes can be stopped and reversed for millions of people, thanks to simple dietary changes and a modest increase in exercise; I'm living proof of that. Experience has shown me that, with the right advice and the right encouragement, we can – every one of us – keep our condition in check. So why isn't this message being heralded by those who govern us? It is a question that makes me angrier than almost any other posed in the modern political arena.

Now that I've come out the other side, relatively unscathed, I believe it's my duty to address this conundrum. It is time for a frank and honest conversation about diabetes in this country, and for radical action to tackle this burgeoning epidemic. My burning ambition, in this context, is to establish a Remission for All movement. A nationwide initiative, propelled by people power, it would be driven by two principal objectives: firstly, to support the estimated 3.4

million UK citizens with type 2 diabetes in trying to regain control of their body and reverse their diagnosis. Secondly, to pressure the government into implementing policy changes that may liberate patients from their condition, and help them to transform their lives. The UK's diabetes crisis is a ticking time-bomb, and we require strong leadership to help us tackle the food corporations, to implement changes to the dietary advice doled out to us and to fund new technology to arm people in their battle against diabetes.

But for so long it's been too easy for the decision-makers to ignore us. So let's make some noise. Let us rise up, join together and form a five-million-strong Remission for All movement – a trade union of diabetics, if you will – to demand the answers and the action that we need. My privileged position means that I can act on others' behalf, not just my own, but I want you to stand up and be counted, too. Because it is only when you speak up, and when we all speak up, that our private tragedies will become a priority for our politicians. We have got to stop feeling guilty, and start getting angry.

Over the past few years, as I've attempted to manage my treatment, I've faced a number of barriers. They certainly aren't unique to me, though. These issues and frustrations are widespread and they are holding diabetics back from getting better. One of the main obstructions faced by type 2 diabetes sufferers, I believe, is a deep-rooted culture of shame. Being diagnosed with T2D is embarrassing. It shouldn't be, but it is. It is wrapped up with a real sense of self-loathing, coupled with a genuine belief that you have brought all this upon yourself, and that you are entirely to blame for the lifestyle choices you've made, the behaviours you've exhibited and the warning signs you've ignored. When you're consumed with so much guilt about your illness, you often find yourself feeling sheepish about asking for the help that you need. Sometimes, your self-esteem is so low that you don't even feel like you deserve that help.

Before I turned my corner, I spent a long time in denial about my diabetes. Like many middle-aged men who are faced with fading youth and failing health, I felt extremely vulnerable. I tried to maintain some kind of equilibrium by managing my illness with drugs and by trying (albeit half-heartedly) to monitor the damage it was doing to me. But I didn't own type 2 diabetes, nor did I fight it; I merely suppressed it. I surrendered to its terrible, inevitable progress. It took me a while to properly understand, and then to fully accept, that I had a life-threatening, life-reducing, life-debilitating condition.

Only after furthering my knowledge with reading and research – especially the work of Dr Michael Mosley and Professor Roy Taylor – did the gravity of this disease begin to hit home. However, while I was able to discuss my subsequent health concerns with Dr Nazeer and Maggie, my diabetes nurse, I was unable to open up to others. I simply couldn't find the inner strength, or the right language, to broach the subject with loved ones. Instead, I continued to carry my guilty little secret around with me, shielding my illness from close friends and family for fear that they'd perceive me as weak-willed and lily-livered. In the cold light of day, I didn't want them to see me how I saw myself: as an abject failure.

The same was true at work. I kept mum about my battle with diabetes in Westminster and West Bromwich, worried that my standing among colleagues, voters and constituents would diminish if news filtered out that I had an illness that was commonly seen as self-inflicted. Society also dictated that MPs should be strong and robust, and wise and responsible, and in my mind, being a diabetes sufferer just didn't fit that mould.

As it transpired, of course, circumstances around my fiftieth birthday prompted me to flick that mental switch and make a stark decision. I was the father of two beautiful children. I was a Member of Parliament. My life ought to have been a joy, not a trial. I could no longer bear the guilt of looking at my son and daughter and thinking that, if I didn't do something, I might not be around to see them off to university, or to take Malachy to the pub for his first pint, or to give Saoirse away at her wedding. I went to war against my own diabetes not only because I wanted to save my own life, but also to be present in my kids' lives.

By now you'll know how I addressed and tackled my type 2 diabetes. And you'll know that my life has been totally transformed as a result. The impact of putting my condition into remission, and regaining my health, has gone far beyond shedding the pounds and sharpening my fitness. I have more energy and enthusiasm. I have a keener focus and a calmer disposition. I enjoy restorative sleep and rejuvenated mornings. Conquering your illness is an exhilarating experience. You discover a new zest for life, and a new zeal for the future. And, soon enough, friends, family and colleagues begin to notice the difference.

'You've become much more kind and considerate since you lost the weight, Tom,' someone very close to me remarked recently. 'You're like a different person, in fact.'

I confess that I look back at some of my 'old self' behaviour with great shame and regret, probably in the same way that a reformed alcoholic reflects upon their days of excess boozing. Had I not been hampered by the double whammy of brain fog and body fatigue, I'd have been able to engage with my family and my colleagues much more meaningfully. With a clearer head, no doubt I could have read more books, and absorbed more knowledge. With more acuity and lucidity, maybe I could have performed better in some elements of my parliamentary work. I recently watched some of my archive Commons performances, and it was truly eye-opening. One in particular – a 2002 intervention demanding better diagnostic tests in sport, with reference to the brain trauma sustained by the late West Brom footballer, Jeff Astle – didn't exactly show me in my best light. It was far too verbose – verging on the rambling, in fact – and it lacked sharpness. As I played it back, I wondered whether I was in the throes of a diabetic 'hypo' that afternoon, due to a dip in my blood glucose levels. One thing's for sure: I'd have definitely headed for the Commons vending machine straight afterwards for my obligatory KitKat Chunky.

*

The revelation of my diagnosis at the ukactive Conference in 2018 (and having also spoken about it earlier on *Good Morning Britain*) proved to be a momentous step on my health journey. The prospect of speaking at the conference concerned me for two reasons. Firstly, by confessing that I was a T2D sufferer, I was publicly revealing something that could be construed as a weakness (not always a good move for a politician); and secondly, by talking about my recovery, I was adding to the diabetes-shaming narrative that places the onus on you to fix yourself post-diagnosis, because you're at fault. As it turned out, opening up about my condition was liberating, and explaining how I'd driven my diabetes into remission unburdened me of a heavy weight. I really needn't have been so nervous, either, since the response from my audience couldn't have been more warm and encouraging.

It is, of course, an intensely personal decision as to whether you openly discuss your own health matters, but, for people in the public eye, I believe such candour can have a hugely positive impact. Just sitting in a TV studio and saying 'Guess what, I'm a type 2 diabetic' can have an amazing ripple effect, in that it can resonate with millions of people across the nation. I would really love to see more high-profile individuals leading the way. Imagine if a world-famous actor or musician was prepared to speak out in public about their experience of living with T2D? It would make it so much easier to have a national debate about various issues that could ultimately save countless lives.

In retrospect, I wished I'd had the courage to open up about my condition sooner, as I might have been able to influence public policy much earlier. But I was so glad that, in the end, I plucked up the courage to say my piece. My ukactive speech, and the ensuing media coverage, unleashed a huge wave of emails containing stories from type 2 diabetes sufferers across the country, some of whom were still battling with the disease and some of whom, like me, had managed to conquer it. Tellingly, and touchingly, I received many messages from men in their forties and fifties without a formal medical diagnosis who, having seen me on the telly, had recognised their own symptoms. As a consequence, they'd been prompted to visit their GP, or to confide in their partners, or both.

Others who'd trodden similar paths to mine got in touch, too.

'Hi Tom,' began one of the emails that hit my inbox that autumn. 'Lots of fellow diabetics want to join you in your plight. We have reversed the condition in exactly the same way. Low carb. It's so exciting to read about your goals. Please count us in. We are here to support you and take forward the cause any way we can. Changes need to happen and the faster the better. Thanks.'

'Well done in your "battle" with type 2 diabetes,' commented the husband of a T2D patient. 'My wife has also done well by sorting out both her diet and her exercise levels. I am really proud of her for her efforts, and I am glad to read of another sufferer who has decided to tackle the problem face-on.'

'Congratulations, Tom! Bravo!' wrote a well-wisher. 'Well done and best wishes for a healthy future. Best thing you've done so far for the British people (and probably the world). For the mass target population (when you're in government) we surely need the food industry to co-operate and almost certainly some amount of legislation (and never mind the misplaced howls of "nanny state" from the usual quarters). All best.'

Once my diagnosis was in the public domain, I soon found myself deploying my ultra-sensitive T2D radar. Sometimes I'd spot a colleague with a telltale clammy face and protruding belly – just as I'd exhibited, back in the day – and would try to find a tactful way in which to broach this most sensitive of issues. I felt compelled to do so; I had developed an almost evangelical desire to get the early-diagnosis message out there.

'Hi mate, how are you doing these days?' I'd ask as we both filed into the Commons voting lobby, purposely initiating a conversation that, I hoped, would be rounded off with a friendly suggestion to perhaps visit a GP, or consider getting a blood test. I couldn't bear the thought of anyone suffering with ill-health, like I'd done for so long.

I grew up in the trade union movement and, since then, every aspect of my politics has been shaped and underpinned by the principles of endeavour and collective action. The power of that movement, after all, was to take what were private and individual tragedies (which were often tinged with shame) and turn them into a shared struggle for justice. Whether it was someone unfairly losing their job, experiencing bullying at work or being paid less due to their gender, these inequities would be addressed and resolved together, in partnership.

I believe that we diabetics ought to take a leaf out of the trade union playbook. We should speak up, in unison, about what we need. That way we will be harder to ignore. That way, too, the personal battle we each face – to obtain the information, the support and the treatment that we require – will be taken out of the private sphere of the doctor's surgery and into the public realm of governance, where the big decisions are made.

Sadly, the political class continue to ignore us. The lazy stereotype of diabetics – that we are fat, indolent and lacking in self-control and self-respect – is a powerful one, and it gives politicians (and occasionally the media) a convenient excuse to turn a blind eye. We are to blame, so the logic goes, and therefore we are never the priority. We are presented as somehow less deserving than those who suffer with other illnesses.

It is this passive disregard that leads to the 'upstream' spending of billions of pounds on the complications of diabetes – the amputations, the strokes, the dementia – that could easily be avoided 'downstream' (I don't think I'm divulging any trade secrets when I confess that we British politicians aren't exactly known for our long-termism, or for our grasp of logic).

But what about intervening much, much earlier?

What about catching people before they fall into illness? Currently, government attention in this area is focused on those presenting with pre-diabetes, whose blood sugar levels are dangerously high, but not so much that they can be diagnosed as diabetics. These people are further back on the timeline to potentially having their feet removed by an NHS surgeon or being treated for impending blindness. Naturally, it's right and proper that we intervene at this stage – I wish that I'd been able to tackle my illness before it developed into full-blown diabetes – but the truth is that we could be starting a whole lot earlier. And in doing so we could be heading diabetes off at the pass for millions of people, before it starts to wreak significant damage. What if we could start addressing nutrition before the pre-diabetes stage?

Years before pre-diabetes, you become obese. That's the trigger; that's the early warning system. So why don't we intervene then? The honest answer from ministers is rationing or, in other words, the controlled distribution of scarce resources. Too many of us are obese for the system to cope. Too many people are heading for diabetes, meaning that government cannot spend the money up front to prevent them reaching that terrible place. Fair enough, I suppose – there isn't infinite cash to splash – but this is such a short-sighted view, even from the depressing vantage point of a bean-counting minister.

My despair and embarrassment about my condition has since catalysed into determination and anger. Determination to get better and to help others to do so, and anger at all those politicians and food manufacturers who get in the way of mass recovery. I am committed to fighting my corner, however. Activism is in my blood. As an MP, I've always been a bit of a rebel with a taste for campaigning. I've resigned from frontbench positions under the last three Labour leaders and I've fought what looked like hopeless campaigns – against the Murdoch empire, for one – and have caused so much trouble for powerful people that at one point I was followed by private investigators who rifled through my bins on a nightly basis (only to find, back then, a lot of empty takeaway containers from the local curry house). Well, I've got a new mission nowadays. To channel my frustrations, and your frustrations, into real action for change. We are going to turn Remission for All into a reality.

I have, as it happens, spent much of the last two years shaking the tree at Westminster. I've become an agitator, an irritant. I have asked awkward parliamentary questions of Conservative ministers (a method by which MPs keep these individuals on their toes, to demonstrate that an issue is important). They have been grilled about the impact of banning the advertising of high-sugar milk products on public transport, for example (the health secretary at the time said he'd not assessed it). They've been asked when the government would consider expanding the sugar levy from fizzy drinks to sweetened milk products (the then chancellor replied that he had no plans to extend it).

I suppose it's a bit like playing political cricket; I'm bowling questions at ministers to expose deficiencies in their thinking, and holes in their strategy. I am keen to maintain the pressure because I cannot think of another policy area – at such a senior level in government – in which a huge problem has received so little bandwidth. And those ministers' answers tell me that our government is still in complacency mode when it comes to our health, and when it comes to our kids' chances of avoiding the same traps that have ensnared previous generations.

Eventually, through questions and scrutiny, you can establish facts that are so strong that ministers are compelled to take action. When I was investigating phone hacking it was the disclosure that journalists had intercepted the phone of a kidnapped schoolgirl that led to the prime minister being forced to act. In the case of type 2 diabetes, I thought my revelation that over 150 diabetes-related amputations are made each week in the UK might gain some traction, and might prompt the government to further resource some targeted prevention programmes. Sadly, although my parliamentary interventions attracted a bit of newspaper coverage, very little changed. It wasn't just type 2 diabetics who ignored their own condition; there was a national collective denial about it, too.

There are many good people working for charities and campaign groups who are trying to support people through type 2 diabetes. Talk to the leaders of these organisations, however, and they'll tell you that the NHS will collapse if the rate of increase in T2D continues to rise. Yet their public demands of government are incremental, when what is needed is a massive step change. Type 2 diabetes is a public health emergency. It requires powerful leadership, a paradigm shift in thinking and the focused attention of legislators, regulators, retailers and food producers. Unfortunately, I fear that the charities that seek to speak for us are captured by the same complacency as our politicians. Many of them lack ambition and urgency. And others – through dodgy deals with PepsiCo, for example – are difficult to trust.

In the spring of 2019 I decided that I needed to stimulate some fresh thinking. I needed to encourage an injection of new ideas that were deliverable, but that were not held back by the 'computer says no' approach shown by many of our health establishments. Taking this into account, I set up a small independent commission, on a shoestring budget, to answer a simple question:

How do we halt the rise of type 2 diabetes over the lifetime of a single parliament?

I was advised not to do it this way, simply because many people think it's impossible to achieve, such is the degradation of our food supply. Yet how long are we going to leave it before we finally admit the game is up? How many more millions of lives do we want to see blighted before we address the root cause of type 2 diabetes, namely our national diet? How long before we confront the big food conglomerates and their army of lobbyists to say that enough is enough? The high prevalence of processed foods and sugar-laden products already means that one in three pupils is leaving primary school overweight or obese, and that more teenagers than ever are being diagnosed with T2D.

I want to include type 2 diabetes as part of the debate at

a general election, and with that in mind I'm hoping that my commission will report its findings in time for the political parties to promise meaningful changes in their manifestos. That's my hope. But the complacency found within our health and political establishment does not fill me with optimism. So I need your help. Five million type 2 diabetics demanding Remission for All would do it, I'm sure.

The tragedy of type 2 diabetes is that, if the research is accurate, at least two million of us can rid ourselves of the condition completely with simple nutritional changes, combined with a slightly more active life. As I discovered myself, when I eradicated takeaways, processed food, refined sugar and starchy carbs – as well as upping my exercise – my blood glucose levels returned to normal, and I no longer needed to be medicated. As a result of this change in diet and behaviour, my own type 2 diabetes went into remission, and I became physically and emotionally energised.

My experience as a type 2 diabetes sufferer has made me think much harder about tackling obesity-related health problems. The first thing we need to do, I reckon, is to scrap once and for all the ridiculous notion that we all share the same behaviours and the same body chemistry. Key to my Remission for All movement would be a call to overhaul the 'one size fits all' dietary guidelines endorsed by the government. Many of us with T2D need to lose weight, but that doesn't mean that we should have to follow a standardised eating plan. This is a simple fact that all doctors and politicians need to get their heads around – I can't stress this enough – because the current passivity about dietary guidance and treatment plans is killing people. A single model of wellness is being adopted by health authorities before being applied to everyone, ignoring the evidence that we all have different bodies, with different biochemistry and with different triggers.

Of the people I know who have put their diabetes in remission, the majority have done so by ignoring Public Health England's controversial Eatwell Guide (the more recent incarnation of the Eatwell Plate). Don't get me wrong, it helped me, to a degree, when I was first diagnosed. It showed me that my carbohydrate intake was off the scale and way beyond the 'normal' range, which helped me limit (but not eliminate) the rice, chips and bread that had formed the basis of a very poor diet.

Many prominent healthcare professionals have since debunked the high-carb, low-fat Eatwell Guide. They have instead advocated a low-carb, low-sugar eating plan as a means of not only losing weight, but also tackling blood glucose issues, with a view to putting type 2 diabetes into remission. Having assiduously researched the subject, I carefully chose to follow a ketogenic nutrition eating plan, the principles of which, no matter how they were interpreted, directly contradicted the Eatwell Guide as regards the amount of carbohydrates a person should consume. But, to me, this regimented diet was a revelation. It enabled me to tackle my sucrose addiction, and it also allowed me to control my eating habits and curb my hunger cravings. The massive weight loss that ensued then liberated me to take up exercise and become more active.

If we're going to really crack this crisis, we need to give bespoke nutritional advice to diabetes sufferers. We should formulate individual eating plans that correspond to a particular patient's requirements, rather than trying to be a catch-all for the whole population. We have to offer customised diets that consider everything we know about nutrition, instead of rigidly adhering to one dietary doctrine that has somehow won through at the top, and is now carved into stone like the Ten Commandments.

Essentially, I believe that we have to ditch the Eatwell Guide as the bible of nutritional advice. I am not saying that it's always wrong – I'm not saying that it's always right, either – but I do feel that its dogmatic use by NHS practitioners is often counterproductive in terms of making people better, especially those with type 2 diabetes. Although abandoning Eatwell might seem a controversial move, I'm pretty sure that most local doctors would be receptive to the idea, particularly if they received training to understand why so many voice their concerns about its inflexibility. I get the distinct impression that most GPs (and medical students, for that matter) simply don't receive adequate training in nutritional science, and as such are left wholly dependent on the unyielding orthodoxy of official advice.

During the Reformation, when Christians across Europe rebelled against the Catholic church, one of the major feuds centred around the claim that priests learned the Bible by rote, without understanding a word it said. They could give you chapter and verse in pretty good Latin, apparently, but didn't really know the story of Jesus, let alone the theology underpinning it. From my experience, discussing nutrition-related issues with general practitioners feels like talking to a pre-Reformation priest about the Holy Trinity. They know the words they're supposed to say, but they don't understand the meaning of it at all.

The Eatwell Guide is loaded with carbohydrates. It advises us to fill up on foodstuffs that are on the ketogenic nutrition 'banned' list. Five years ago, I'd have never suspected that the spaghetti carbonara that I regularly piled onto my plate was one of the worst meals for me to consume. And, what's more, the Eatwell Guide would have left me none the wiser. For people like me, with type 2 diabetes, this advice is not just unhelpful; it's downright dangerous. As far as I'm concerned, telling T2D patients to eat pasta in order to become healthier is like telling an alcoholic to drink vodka because it doesn't taste like alcohol.

When I shed all my weight, I experienced a host of conflicting emotions. On the one hand, I felt exhilarated to have reclaimed my good health and to have ditched my XXXL T-shirts. On the other hand, I felt angry and frustrated about the way I'd had to tackle my obesity. I shouldn't have had to join the dots myself. I shouldn't have had to ignore my own government's nutritional guidelines to get myself well. I shouldn't have had to feel guilty for putting beautiful grass-fed butter into my coffee. And I certainly could have done without BOGOFs on crappy processed food when I was doing my weekly shop. And all that was before I witnessed 'Big Sugar' firms blatantly targeting young children in the UK, even before they reached primary school. That's when my anger *really* turned to rage.

In the previous chapter, I discussed how our choices and options have been engineered in order to push us into obesity and diabetes. We are not solely responsible for the junk food that we eat or the sugary pop that we drink. It is almost impossible for people to keep the weight off when the system is stacked against them, and I am sick to the gills of tabloids and politicians continually knocking and judging the overweight.

It is not our fault that we have developed type 2 diabetes. Our chances of getting better massively depend on the support and guidance that we are given. While it may well be within our power to improve our health, our lifestyle and our longevity, this doesn't mean that the onus should rest on us to do it on our own. We need food manufacturers, retailers, policymakers and politicians to work together to make it easier for people to eat more healthily and get more exercise.

This is one of the reasons why I think Remission for All is a necessity, as it would encourage a national debate about diet and nutrition issues for those suffering with type 2 diabetes, or those susceptible to the condition. Sitting behind the current quota of 3.4 million type 2 diabetics, you see, are another million undiagnosed type 2 diabetics. And sitting behind them are over 12 million people who are at risk of the disease. As families and communities – and as a country – we simply cannot afford the personal or financial cost of that potential increase.

It is quite clear to me that we need to challenge those clinicians whose default position is to offer prescription drugs as the first-line treatment for type 2 diabetes patients (as well as those pharmaceutical firms who may have financial motivations for medicalising us). Indeed, I do believe that we've now reached the stage where every GP in the land should receive specific diet and nutrition training, to enable them to offer patient-centred guidance for those diagnosed with T2D. It is time to adopt a far more holistic approach, and to promote a deeper sense of partnership between doctor and patient. It is my understanding that many GPs feel tethered to the Eatwell edict, and – for fear of being reported to official bodies, and jeopardising their professional careers – are deterred from offering conflicting advice. As a result, they are still having to recommend carbohydrate-heavy diet pro-grammes to their T2D patients, promoting the consumption of the very foodstuffs that played havoc with my own insulin levels.

There do exist, fortunately, some forward-thinking GPs who are bucking the trend. These progressive practitioners are freely advocating low-carb, high-fat diets as a way of preventing and managing T2D, the ultimate aim being to reduce the need for heavy medication and to maximise the likelihood of remission. Among their number is Southportbased Dr David Unwin, the self-styled 'Low Carb GP', who has become something of a legendary figure in the world of diabetes. His bespoke Low Carb Program has seen extraordinary results, with many of his patients putting their T2D into remission, which, as a consequence, has had a transformational effect upon their lives. His message is a simple one, based upon simple recommendations that many dieticians would concur with. In order to lose weight and regain their good health, Dr Unwin believes, patients with type 2 diabetes need to cut down on sugary food and starchy carbs and need to increase their intake of leafy green vegetables.

It took the counter-intuitive, revolutionary inventiveness of this pioneering Merseyside GP to demonstrate just how badly carbohydrates affected me, in the starkest of terms. His team set up a study to examine the glycaemic index of commonly eaten foods (the GI being the level at which food raises blood glucose levels), before converting that figure into its equivalent in teaspoons-worth of sugar. They discovered that a portion of basmati rice – one of my staple foods when I was 22 stone (140 kilos) – had a GI equal to ten teaspoons of sugar. So, over a lifetime of rice-eating, I worked out that I'd consumed a total of 39,000 teaspoons of sugar, which amounted to 390 kilos of the stuff. Even more worryingly, this was possibly a conservative estimate. No wonder I spent years experiencing sudden spikes in blood glucose levels.

In 2018, Dr Unwin's GP practice saved nearly £60,000 on drugs for conditions including hypertension and type

2 diabetes through, in his words, his 'passion for offering patients the alternative of lifestyle medicine and support'. His weekly graphs – which demonstrate how his patients' HbA1c levels are impacted when they link their diet to the glycaemic index – should be the envy of every GP. I truly believe that his credo is the way forward and, in an ideal world, should be rolled out to every health centre in the country. It works, it costs virtually nothing and it saves the NHS tons of money further down the line.

Best of all, medics like Dr Unwin give people like me their lives back. Yes, I have to make do without my beloved basmati rice, and I'm sorry for the damage this has done to my local curry house's bottom line, but it's a price that I'm more than willing to pay.

So we know that the current guidance doesn't work and that we can do so much better for those with a type 2 diagnosis. We know that people need individual, personalised advice rather than a one-size-fits-all axiom. And we know that more GPs need to be trained properly in nutritional science so that their patients can benefit from the latest research. There are, however, other cost-effective measures and technological advances that may be game-changers, insofar as they can improve the health of individuals, and can also save some money for our beleaguered NHS.

According to a good friend of mine, a diabetes nurse, a gadget called a continuous glucose monitor represents the greatest advance in diabetes treatment for a quarter of a century. CGMs allow patients to monitor how their body responds to food by indicating which products cause a spike in blood sugar. If obesity is the air raid siren for diabetes, then a CGM is the radar, allowing individuals to track, in real time, how they react to certain foodstuffs. These nifty devices are currently prescribed for type 1 diabetics on the NHS, for the obvious reason that they are potential lifesavers. But their capacity goes far beyond that. In my view, relatively soon they'll replace the finger-prick testing kits currently used by many type 2 diabetics.

I actually tested out a CGM monitor for two weeks while researching for this book. They're incredible contraptions, although I had to force-feed myself some chocolate Hobnobs in order to ascertain how my body responded to a sugar injection. Not particularly well, was the answer, although it wasn't nearly as bad as I was expecting. What this CGM gave me, however, was the acquisition of much more granular data. Knowing that biscuit X raised my blood sugars to level Y put me in charge of my body, and gave me a certain ownership. Anyone who has struggled to lose weight and manage their diabetes will know that this feeling of self-control is all too rare during that lonely, difficult battle.

But testing the CGM also made me feel somewhat maudlin, to be honest. It made me feel quite sorry for the 30-year-old me, Tom version 1.0, the podgy bloke with a spiralling sugar addiction. If I'd had a CGM monitor at my disposal following a Friday night of lager and curry — particularly after guzzling a two-litre bottle of Coke the morning after – I'd have experienced a blood sugar spike of Himalayan proportions. By understanding my own data in these extreme circumstances, I think I might have addressed my nutrition earlier, perhaps even before I'd broken myself enough to develop diabetes.

A fully functioning Remission for All movement would definitely include a call for every obese person to be given a continuous glucose monitor on the NHS. I reckon they'd only need to use them for a few weeks before they'd begin to comprehend the damaging impact of high-sugar, highly processed food upon their general health. The CGM might then provide the impetus for these poorly individuals to kick-start a new diet and fitness regime, which could prompt them to lose some weight, alter their lifestyle and ultimately ditch their medication. The NHS (and us taxpayers) would be much better off, too. Yet another win-win situation.

As I write this book, however, I can't see anyone in power calling for this fabulous piece of technology to be deployed and distributed in this manner. This frustrates and infuriates me. We are allowing people to get ill, and to ultimately die, because we aren't being ambitious or imaginative enough about new technology that may arm us in our fight against obesity and poor nutrition.

On Monday 10 June 2019 I hit my eight-stone (51-kilo) weight-loss target, just under two years after commencing my diet and fitness plan. This milestone occurred in the midst of the Brexit crisis in parliament, possibly the most stressful stage in my career to date; I'd never known such pressures of work at Westminster and, as deputy leader, had never experienced so many demands on my time. Though delighted to have shed every single one of those 112 pounds – I couldn't quite believe that I'd done it – I found myself being dogged by a deeper, existential question.

If I hadn't lost that eight stone, would I still be alive today?

In all honesty, and without being melodramatic, I think I've dodged a bullet. I genuinely do. Looking back to the summer of 2017, when I ate too much food and did too little exercise, I reckon I was weeks or months away from having a heart attack. Had I not decided to ring the changes when I did, I think I'd have definitely keeled over at some point. I can't see how I could have carried on dealing with my chock-full diary and my ever-increasing workload without having some kind of physical breakdown. I have no intention of returning to that state of affairs, of course. In fact, I'd rather give up my role in politics – which I adore – than lose my health. My life is just too precious to even think about downing a Coke or devouring a pizza.

Speaking of which, toward the end of 2019 I achieved another milestone. I finally hit the 'unsubscribe' button on the emails sent to me by my local pizza delivery service. All those 2-for-1 deals, money-off vouchers and free delivery offers that had seduced me for years were finally consigned to history. For a while I'd just ignored them – I was perversely satisfied by the fact that I had the willpower to do so – but the time soon came for me to delete them for ever. And, you know what? It felt absolutely bloody brilliant.

I live in hope that, one day, there'll be millions of other type 2 diabetes sufferers who, having transformed their lives through diet and exercise, will also find themselves zapping those fast-food outlets from their inboxes. I want them to experience that same sense of satisfaction. I want them to be proud of their accomplishments. I want them to go on to live a life free of guilt, and full of joy. And then I want them to join forces with me in promoting a hugely important message.

Remission. For all.

Epilogue

There are occasions, as a politician, when a single statistic can stop you in your tracks. It was while attending an event at the House of Commons in the spring of 2019 that I found myself chatting with the CEO of the Outdoor Industries Association, a group that lobbies parliament on behalf of such organisations as British Cycling, National Parks, Ramblers and the Canal & River Trust. Andrew Denton was an impressive character – in his spare time he was a triathlete, mountaineer and paraglider – and it was while discussing some government-related issues that he shared a jaw-dropping stat.

'Did you know, Tom, that three-quarters of kids in this country spend less time outdoors than high-security prisoners?' he said, referring to a 2016 survey that had identified that 74 per cent of children played in the open air for under an hour per day (an hour being the daily norm for inmates) and, furthermore, that one in five youngsters never spent any leisure time outside whatsoever.

'My God, how appalling,' I said. 'That's nothing short of a national tragedy.'

Our conversation played on my mind for days. Not only had Andrew's words challenged me as a policymaker, they had, perhaps more deeply, challenged me as a parent.

While my son and daughter spent a decent amount of time outdoors (Malachy loved running around the gym and Saoirse was a keen netballer), I still had fatherly concerns about the number of hours they spent watching Netflix and playing on consoles. Were my kids too reliant on screens for their entertainment? Was I doing enough to encourage them into the great outdoors? Did we visit enough of our country's beautiful parks, forests and beaches?

The following week I set up a meeting with Andrew to discuss the problem of these confined lifestyles.

'You really made me stop and think the other day, Andrew,' I said. 'So much so, in fact, that I'd like to start work on an outdoor recreation policy, as part of my remit for sport. Something for the next Labour Party manifesto, maybe.'

I told him how I wanted to help encourage everyone in the UK, young or old, to have more active lifestyles without breaking the bank, and how I wanted to work in tandem with groups and organisations to improve access to outdoor pursuits.

'Yeah, that all sounds very interesting, Tom,' replied Andrew, slowly nodding his head.

'But what would be really great,' I added, 'would be if you could get on board in some way. Help me to set up a consultation, perhaps, or put me in touch with a few of your contacts in the industry. I doubt anyone knows more about these issues than you.'

'Okay, now please don't take this the wrong way' – he sighed – 'but do you know how many similar conversations

I've had with politicians, of all persuasions? Dozens. And nothing ever comes of them. Nothing. Let's just say that, over time, I've become a little cynical.'

Well, that was me put in my place.

'Listen, I get where you're coming from,' he continued, 'but I'd only be prepared to help you with this if you walk the walk, not just talk the talk. If you're going to practise what you preach, you'll need to sample the great outdoors yourself. I mean, when was the last time you climbed a hill?'

I paused to think for a moment.

'When I was in the Scouts, I reckon.'

'My point exactly.' He smiled.

In the space of an hour, the persuasive Mr Denton had convinced me to take part in a quartet of outdoor challenges that would span a period of six months: climbing Snowdon in mid-Wales, kayaking along a network of canals in the West Midlands, cycling the 46-mile (74-kilometre) Prudential RideLondon and tackling a half-mile open-water swim in the Serpentine. We came up with the idea of grouping them all into an '#Adventures4Health' initiative that would see me joining forces with the OIA (and ukactive, its umbrella organisation) to promote the benefits of outdoor recreation and helping them to raise the media profile of each event.

Tom, what on earth are you letting yourself in for? said a little voice in my head.

'An absolute pleasure doing business with you,' said a grinning Andrew, vigorously shaking my hand.

Though I'd never been in better shape health-wise, the prospect of these physical challenges gave me the collywobbles. I could barely swim, I hadn't been up a mountain for three decades, I'd never been in a canoe (cramming myself into a seaside dinghy was the nearest I'd got) and I was still a little unsteady on my bicycle. #Adventures4Health was way beyond my comfort zone, and would prove more challenging than anything I'd done hitherto.

That said, Andrew's comments were spot on. If I wanted to shape policy to help others explore the UK's green spaces, and to find an activity that they enjoyed, it was down to me to set a good example. By speaking openly about my own backstory – how a middle-aged fat bloke lost weight and got active – I would hopefully strike a chord with others in similar predicaments.

'Through #Adventures4Health, I want to show other people what is possible as an individual and how easy it is to access so many different activities, in every part of the country,' I stated in the OIA press release. 'We face a growing inactivity epidemic in the UK and it's killing people, but it doesn't have to be this way.'

Over this half-year period I'd also be raising funds for four different charities: the Albion Foundation (West Bromwich Albion FC's community scheme); SpecialEffect (an organisation that uses video games to enhance the lives of disabled people); Lumos (an NGO founded by J. K. Rowling that promotes an end to the institutionalisation of children around the world); and the Cystic Fibrosis Trust, which funds research into therapies and treatments to help those with the condition live longer and healthier lives. All four causes were very close to my heart, and many of my friends, colleagues and family members were kind enough to donate to my fundraising webpage.

'Two years ago, if you'd have asked me who'd be a hundred pounds lighter and climbing Snowdon, you would have been last on the list,' said Dave Ashlee, my old mate from school.

The first of the four challenges, the trek up Snowdon (or Yr Wyddfa), took place on Saturday 18 May. As an experienced hiker and climber, Andrew Denton had given me plenty of advice beforehand to ensure that I was well-prepared and well-equipped. Sturdy, ankle-supporting footwear was essential, as was a decent waterproof and layers of extra-warm clothing (not forgetting a flask and a lunchbox). While Snowdon was one of the most accessible and enjoyable mountains to scale – thousands did so each year – every climber had to have their wits about them. Weather conditions on the peak were unpredictable, even in spring and summer, and the environment could easily become treacherous. 'Four seasons in one day' commonly occurred on Snowdon, which often meant starting the ascent on a warm and sunny morning, yet still meeting thick clouds and plummeting temperatures as you reached the summit.

Our 20-strong climbing party stayed overnight at the Plas y Brenin National Outdoor Centre, waking up at 4.30 a.m. to catch the minibus to the foot of the mountain (by arriving earlier, we hoped to avoid the weekend throng). As we drew nearer, and I caught sight of the summit dominating the skyline, I could barely believe this was happening. Eighteen months previously I'd struggled to get up a stepladder, let alone a mountain, yet I now found myself preparing to tackle the highest peak in England and Wales (the site of Sir Edmund Hillary's pre-Everest training, no less).

In our group that morning, other than Andrew and some industry representatives, were members of my Westminster team, including my parliamentary assistants Jo Dalton, Sarah Coombes, Haf Davies, Danny Adilypour and Nicole Trehy. It was something of a cross-party affair, too, since also joining us that day was the Conservative MP for Wyre Forest, Mark Garnier, and his wife Caroline.

'How are you feeling, Tom?' he asked as we assembled at the starting point.

'Nerves are starting to kick in a bit,' I replied. 'Fear of the unknown, I reckon...'

We were accompanied by an experienced guide, Jason Rawles, who had kindly agreed to donate his time and his vast experience to keep us safe on the ascent. We took the Pyg track, which is considered one of the easier-to-follow paths and so was well suited to those, like me, with limited hill-walking experience. Nevertheless, the first few hundred metres of the climb were incredibly tough going – the incline was steep, and the terrain was rugged – and, as I dug in my heels, and inhaled the thin air, I could feel panic starting to rise.

I'm not so sure I can make it to the top, I thought, as I puffed and panted up the rocky path.

'You're doing great, Tom,' said Andrew, hanging back from the front of the group, and falling into step with me. 'It levels out soon, I promise.'

Indeed, for the next couple of hours the intensity of the slog relented and, as I finally relaxed into the climb, I even took the opportunity to rekindle my love of Ordnance Survey maps. I could vaguely remember how to navigate using an OS and a compass – I'd done a spot of orienteering in my teenage years – and really enjoyed deciphering the map symbols and figuring out the grid references.

'It's a lot easier navigating this than Brexit, that's for sure,' I said to Nick Giles, the MD of Ordnance Survey, who had come on the climb with us and had despatched a few handy hints and tips along the way. I also found myself having a great chat with Simon McGrath, Communications Director of the Camping and Caravanning Club, who got me thinking about investing in a second-hand campervan one day in the future and travelling around the UK's glorious coastline every weekend.

As the final ascent began, however, via a long, steep and arduous incline, my capacity for conversation diminished. We had been climbing for almost three hours and my energy levels started to dip; instead of chatting, for the last stretch I concentrated solely on my breathing and my footing.

It was around 10.30 a.m. that the group finally reached Snowdon's majestic summit, 1,085 metres above sea level. My first #Adventures4Health challenge had been completed. It felt tremendous to conquer this giant of a mountain, and to achieve this personal milestone, and there were many whoops, hugs and selfies as #TeamSnowdon celebrated our feat.

'So when are we tackling Ben Nevis and Scafell Pike, then?' I asked Jo as we headed to the Summit Café for a much-needed refuel. My tweet later that day summed up my feeling of euphoria.

> @tom_watson
>
> Two years ago – aged 50, weighing 22 stone, with T2 diabetes – climbing to the summit of Snowdon was unfathomable. Today, 100lb lighter and in remission from T2, I've done it. Thank you everyone for your amazing support and inspiration.

The second component of my #Adventures4Health challenge – the kayak paddle, in partnership with British Canoeing – took place two months later, on Saturday 20 July. The plan was to wind my way down a nine-mile (14.5-kilometre) stretch of waterways in my native West Midlands, commencing in Tipton and culminating in Birmingham city centre. As the event drew nearer, I took some time out to promote the 'Clear Access, Clear Water' campaign. An initiative spearheaded by British Canoeing, in conjunction with key stakeholders like the Canal & River Trust and the Inland Waterways Association, it called for cleaner, healthier waters, and championed increased public access to our amazing 'blue' spaces. Nine million UK citizens live within a five-minute walk of these waterways – there are more canals in the Black Country than in Venice, believe it or not – but only 4 per cent of waterways are open to canoeists since, on the whole, they flow through privately owned land.

The challenge itself was more toilsome than I'd expected. There was no current on the canal to buffet me along, and I was faced with a stiff breeze and a steady drizzle. However, thanks to the previous week's practice session with British Canoeing, I managed to stay afloat without capsizing. Encouraging me mile by mile were my fellow paddlers, a diverse group that included novices like me as well as elite athletes like Lizzie Broughton, a world champion canoe sprinter; I could only watch in awe as she effortlessly glided through the water, barely causing a ripple (unlike my rather splash-happy self).

As I weaved my way through my West Bromwich constituency I passed countless joggers and dog-walkers on the towpath. They included an elderly lady with a Border collie, who looked on with amusement as her bedraggled MP lifted a kayak over a canal lock.

'Good morning, Mr Watson,' she said. 'Having fun?'

'I think so,' I said with a smile, before scrambling back into the kayak.

Around the halfway stage, my son Malachy, together with his good friends Ned, Frank and Oscar, donned their life jackets and safety helmets and joined our flotilla. It had taken some cajoling the previous day to persuade them to take part (these teenagers were way too cool to canoe) but, as it happened, he and his pals had a whale of a time doing something a little different with their

Saturday. Just before lunchtime, we arrived to a warm welcome at our final destination, Birmingham's Brindleyplace complex (named after genius canal engineer James Brindley, and home to the Malt House pub where, during the 1998 G8 Summit, Tony Blair had bought Bill Clinton a pint).

Completing this three-and-a-half-hour paddle – armachingly gruelling though it was – may not have provoked the same sense of euphoria as climbing Snowdon. That didn't mean that I felt any less proud of myself, however, for clambering into a kayak and testing my mettle.

A week or so later, I found myself back on the water. I had caught the kayaking bug – I'd loved the peace and tranquillity of it all – and when my mate John, an amateur canoeist, had invited me to join him I'd leapt at the chance.

'It's a lovely evening, Tom…' he'd texted after work one Friday. 'Fancy a paddle down the Severn?'

'You betcha,' I'd replied.

With his second-hand, two-man craft strapped onto the roof of his car, my mate and I headed off to Arley, a quaint riverside village near Kidderminster, before spending an idyllic couple of hours messing about on the river while reminiscing about eighties music, all against the backdrop of a mellow summer sunset.

Spending quality time in the great outdoors altered my whole perspective on fitness and exercise, and led to a certain change of heart. Back in London, I'd still been attending the upmarket gym in Mayfair and was nearing the end of my intensive 12-week weight training programme. Having benefited so much from the Snowdon climb and the Midlands paddle, though – on a physical, mental and social level – I soon realised that indoor iron-pumping was nowhere near as enjoyable. Working out in the gym was a largely solitary endeavour, taking place in a high-pressure environment, and I often found it a little dull and monotonous. To be frank, I think an element of vanity had taken over, too. Buoyed by my 'transformation', I'd become a tad obsessed with the pursuit of looking better and feeling stronger, and had been seduced by the lure of a swanky gym. The weight training had helped me lose over a stone in two months, granted, but I didn't feel that this schedule was sustainable in the long term. Not only did it sap far too much of my time and money, the associated four-meals-a-day diet regime had become increasingly difficult to implement. All the measuring was an onerous responsibility, even for me, on quite a disciplined nutritional programme anyway, and it just wasn't as enjoyable as cycling in and out of a keto diet.

So I decided to stop attending the posh gym, for fear of turning into a shallow, self-obsessed London luvvie. There were no hard feelings with the staff – they were superb at what they did, and I genuinely appreciated their expert tuition – but it just wasn't for me any more. I would still work with weights (albeit on a much smaller scale, at a much cheaper venue) but would now place much more emphasis on outdoor, health-by-stealth recreational pursuits. I would instead burn up those calories by walking up a hill for five miles, with the sun on my skin, fresh air in my lungs, a friend by my side and nature all around.

Within two weeks of the paddling challenge, on Sunday 4 August, I was preparing to cycle the Prudential RideLondon. Attracting thousands of cyclists of all abilities every year, this hugely popular event was one component of a weekend-long festival of amateur and professional cycling, which saw eight miles of the capital's roads being cordoned off to make them totally, blissfully, traffic-free.

To say that I was nervous, however, was an under-statement. If truth be told, I was absolutely bricking it. The whole ride was being broadcast on TV, there'd be thousands of spectators on the sidelines, and the potential for the public humiliation of a prominent politician going arse-over-tit on his bike was huge (I still had nightmares about catapulting myself into a thicket of nettles). That week I'd not done as much pre-ride training as I'd have liked, either, since there'd been a raft of Brexit-related crises at Westminster. However, I did manage to shoehorn in a couple more Bikeability sessions. I had never really mastered my new bicycle's gears, especially when going uphill, so asked the instructor to explain, in the simplest of terms, the difference between the big cog and the little cog.

'When you're approaching an incline, Tom, you have to move down the gears by using the shifter on the handlebars,' he said, demonstrating on his own bike. 'This then moves the chain to a different cog, and you'll find there's a lot less resistance.'

'Ah, I get it,' I said, as the penny finally dropped.

On the morning of the ride I fuelled up with a supersized full English breakfast, and glugged down plenty of water, before heading out to Queen Elizabeth Olympic Park in east London. The weather was perfect – warm and sunny, with a gentle breeze – and I felt a frisson of excitement every time I spotted a fellow cyclist sporting a race number on their back. At around 10 a.m. I met my pals James and Mark at the starting line, as well as a colleague of mine, Ruth Cadbury MP, who was the chair of our parliamentary cycling group. While all three were far more experienced in the saddle than me (they'd each completed similar 'sportives' in the past), they promised to ride alongside me for the entire course, which I really appreciated.

As our little group wound our way through Canary Wharf, and then Hyde Park, my friends handed me energy gels and protein bars (so that's what those little back pockets on cycling tops were used for) and, whenever they noticed me struggling up a hill, despite my much-improved gear control, they offered me some welcome words of encouragement.

'C'mon Tom,' said my pal James. 'Work those calves…'

'Doing my best, mate,' I panted.

There was plenty of support from the spectators on the sidelines, too (one boisterous group virtually willed me up a steep hill in Wimbledon) and a fair few people spotted me along the route. About halfway through the ride, another cyclist – a forty-something guy sporting a Motor Neurone Disease Association T-shirt – pedalled over.

'Great to see you, Tom,' he said. 'I had to come over to say hi. If it wasn't for you, I wouldn't be doing this today. I read an interview you did last year, which shocked me into sorting out my own diabetes. I'm in remission now. Can't thank you enough.'

'That's brilliant, mate,' I grinned. 'Enjoy the rest of the ride.'

The last leg of the challenge saw our little peloton cycling past Parliament Square, where hundreds of people had gathered to cheer on the riders. Ruth and I couldn't help but laugh when we caught sight of this. In our day job we were accustomed to this large expanse of grass being overrun with Leave and Remain protesters wielding loudhailers, haranguing passing MPs and disrupting media broadcasts. On this occasion, however, the vibe had changed completely.

It was at the junction of Horse Guards Road and the Mall, with fifty metres of the ride remaining, that I caught a glimpse of Malachy and Saoirse, standing on the corner with their gran. Their cries of 'Go, Dad, go!!!' were ringing in my head as I crossed the finish line, feeling exhausted but exultant.

My final #Adventures4Health challenge – a half-mile open swim – promised to be the most punishing task of all. Swim Serpentine, organised by London Marathon Events to raise money for the charity Children With Cancer, was arranged for the morning of Saturday 21 September. As with the cycle ride, my preparation had been somewhat limited. The Brexit situation at Westminster, including Boris Johnson's proroguing of parliament, had been all-consuming and, save a few lengths of the pool during a week-long summer break in Spain, I'd hardly swum a stroke.

I had managed to get my hands on a few related books, however, which introduced me to a subculture of open-water swimming that I never knew existed. One of them – *Pondlife: A Swimmer's Journal* by writer and poet Al Alvarez – was particularly brilliant, detailing as it did this elderly gent's invigorating, all-weather swims in various pools and ponds around the north London suburb of Hampstead.

'The water was just above freezing, the wind howled, the rain stung my face when I swam on my back,' he wrote after one such dip. 'I came out feeling wonderful.'

As things transpired, though – and much to my disappointment – I was unable to tackle the Serpentine swim that Saturday morning. I had to rush down to the Labour Party conference in Brighton much earlier than anticipated, faced with a crisis that required my urgent attention. The event organisers were very sympathetic, however, and I pledged to undertake the swim when it next came around.

Between May and September, I'd experienced three diverse challenges, each with their own set of demands. But it happened to be another event that summer that left the deepest emotional impact. The third annual RunForJo – set up in memory of my friend and colleague, the late MP Jo

Cox – took place on Sunday 23 June at Oakwell Hall and Country Park, in her former constituency of Batley and Spen in West Yorkshire. My lack of fitness had prevented me from taking part in the two previous events (I couldn't have even walked the 2.5-km family fun run, never mind jogged it) but, this time around, I was delighted to enrol. It was a case of being more willing than ready, though. I had never tackled an organised run in my life, so had no idea how I'd fare. I would, however, have my very own running mate to spur me on.

'Dad, can I do the RunForJo with you?' Saoirse had asked a few weeks previously, extremely keen to get involved in this worthy event.

'Of course you can,' I replied. 'You can be my pacemaker.'

I had to really steel myself as I drove through Jo's home town of Batley that morning, with both Saoirse and Malachy in the car (my son had come along to offer moral support). In 2015 I'd campaigned with Jo on those very streets and doorsteps, when she was first running for parliament. This particular constituency was by no means a nailed-on hold for Labour but, as we visited community centres and chatted with residents, I was convinced that this impressive young woman was the ideal candidate. Highly intelligent, innately compassionate and in possession of a warm and sunny disposition, Jo attracted a string of admirers wherever she went.

Jo will go far, I remember thinking to myself as I watched her campaigning that day, winning over locals with her effortless charm. A natural-born parliamentarian...

In the ensuing general election, Labour held the Batley and Spen seat, with Jo gaining an increased majority. It was nothing less than she deserved, I told her when I rang to offer my congratulations.

Just over a year later this wonderful human being was dead, murdered by a right-wing extremist during her constituency surgery in Birstall. It was the worst day of my political life.

Arriving at Oakwell Park that Sunday morning, I felt supercharged with emotion. The previous afternoon, on what would have been her forty-fifth birthday, I'd organised a 'Great Get Together' picnic at Dartmouth Park in West Bromwich, where a large group of us, including fellow MP Liam Byrne, had celebrated Jo's life and work (hundreds of other similar events in her name were taking place across the UK, too). While it had been an inspiring and uplifting occasion, it had made me realise how much Jo was missed, not just by her friends and family, but by the world of politics in general. In her maiden speech to parliament, she'd maintained that 'we have more in common than that which divides us.' Those words had become more powerful than ever before.

Experiencing the carnival atmosphere and the community ethos at the RunForJo event helped to lift my spirits, though. Everywhere I turned people were beaming with happiness – toddlers, teenagers, parents, grandparents – and the organisers had laid on an array of street food and kids' entertainers. Jo's sister Kim, a qualified personal trainer, even led a pre-race warm-up on the main field, encouraging us all to move our bodies to some cheesy eighties tunes. Malachy stood on the perimeter, pointing and laughing as he watched his dad and sister throwing some serious shapes.

The family run started at 11 a.m. It wasn't easy, by any stretch – the ground underfoot was muddy and boggy, and much of the route was uphill – but any discomfort I felt was outweighed by a deep sense of pride. For the first time in my life I was taking part in a community run, and positively buzzed off all the warmth and camaraderie. And, best of all, I found myself jogging alongside my beloved daughter, sharing in that fun, fresh air and freedom that only outdoor activity could give you. I only wished I'd done all this a decade earlier, of course – all those wasted years I'd spent slumped on the sofa slurping cans of cola – but this was not the time for any lingering regret.

That was then, Tom, I thought to myself as I jogged past Oakwell Hall. *This is now.*

I was pleasantly surprised with my performance (no wheezes, no pit-stops) and, as Saoirse and I crossed the finishing line together, holding hands, I found myself overcome with emotion. I shed a tear or two, I'm not ashamed to admit it.

'Go, Team Watson!' yelled Malachy, capturing our moment on his phone's camera.

Within days, I'd printed and framed that snapshot, and had put it on my House of Commons office desk, in pride of place. The photograph wasn't just a memento of how far I'd come on my weight-loss journey, though. Taken by my son,

and featuring my daughter, it was also a lasting reminder of
why I'd embarked upon it in the first place.

Acknowledgements

As Aristotle would probably have said, you make your own luck in life. If I'd turned down a 5am start to be interviewed by ITV's Susanna Reid about Type 2 diabetes, she would not have suggested I write a book about my health journey. Without her interview, the fabulously talented literary agent (and Good Morning Britain viewer), Rory Scarfe might not have been curious enough to pick up the phone to me.

When Rory phoned he suggested I tell my eating and health story. He teamed me up with the remarkably talented and ever patient co-writer Jo Lake, without whom this book would not exist. To this triumvirate of talent, I will be forever grateful.

And double thanks go to Rory and his team at The Neil Blair Partnership for introducing Jo and I to Kyle Books. Judith Hannam, Joanna Copestick, Caroline Brown and the whole team were incredibly supportive throughout, even when the chaotic world of politics screwed up deadlines.

I couldn't have got fit without the advice of Clayton, Nic and Jay, three experienced fitness professionals who taught me a huge amount as I moved from park bench press-up to gym bench chest press. I am very fortunate to have been given an understanding of the wider fitness industry by the good people at UK Active, the organisation that seeks to spread the joy of good health and fitness to everyone in the UK. Thanks to Huw Edwards, Tanni Grey-Thompson and the team for their advice on policy. And to Andrew Denton at the Outdoor Industries Association, thank you for your advice on peddling, paddling and rock hopping. You are an inspiration. Every time I visit the gym I hear the voice of Phil Wood in my head. It's more than 40 years since he taught me PE but like all the very best teachers, he's still making a difference.

The changes I needed to make would not have happened without reading and listening to an array of clinicians, scientists, writers and biohackers, many of whom will never know what a profound impact they have had on my life. Special thanks go to my GP Dr Shaukat Nazeer, Clare Nasir, Max Wind Cowie, Dr Michael Mosley, Dr Matthew Walker, Dr Aseem Malhotra, Dr Jeff Volek, Dr Stephen Phinney, Dave Asprey and Peter Attia MD.

I couldn't have found the time to get fit without the support and flexibility of my team in Westminster: Alicia Kennedy, Sarah Coombes, Haf Davies, Barbara Hearn, Nicole Trehy and former team members, Jo Dalton, Danny Adilypour, James Robinson, Dominic Murphy, Clare Cole, Tom Hamilton and Sarah Goulbourne. My West Bromwich team, who looked on in amazement, were similarly supportive, particularly Kim Frazer and Simon Hackett who never thought they'd see me leaping over gates and running up garden paths.

I have a message to the men of a certain age with whom I enjoy a friendly rivalry involving daily step and weight measurements, run lengths, cycle distances, pool distances and general health banter. Steve Torrance, James Gurling, David Wild, Michael Dugher, Bill Thomas, Dave Ashlee, Dan Watson, Chris Jenkinson and Conrad Bourne, all I can say is try a bit harder tomorrow.

I got fit to live longer for Malachy and Saoirse. Thank you to them and Siobhan for their love and support. And thanks also to Sarah, Gabriel, Rafa and Manny for their humour, encouragement and expert advice on socks and waterproofs.

My final thanks go to the many hundreds of people who have either written, emailed, tweeted or stopped me in the street to give encouragement and feedback. You have been and remain my inspiration.